HEALTH AND OBESITY

Health and Obesity

Editors

Peter T. Kuo, M.D.
Professor of Medicine
Chief, Cardiovascular Diseases
University of Medicine and Dentistry of New Jersey
Rutgers Medical School
Piscataway, New Jersey

Hadley L. Conn, Jr., M.D.
Professor and Chairman
Department of Medicine
University of Medicine and Dentistry
of New Jersey
Rutgers Medical School
Piscataway, New Jersey

Eugene A. DeFelice, M.D.
Clinical Associate Professor of Medicine
University of Medicine and Dentistry
of New Jersey
Rutgers Medical School
Piscataway, New Jersey

Raven Press ■ New York

Raven Press, 1140 Avenue of the Americas, New York, New York 10036

Library of Congress Cataloging in Publication Data
Main entry under title:

Health and obesity.

    Includes bibliographies and index.
    1. Obesity.   2. Health.   I. Conn, Hadley L.
II. DeFelice, Eugene A.   III. Kuo, Peter T. [DNLM:
1. Obesity—Congresses.   WD 210 H434 1981]
RC628.H4 1983   616.3'98   82-12295
ISBN 0-89004-809-6

Made in the United States of America

Introduction

I am pleased to introduce this volume which is based on the proceedings of the Health and Obesity symposium sponsored by the University of Medicine and Dentistry of New Jersey-Rutgers Medical School. Publications of this kind are a major responsibility of a public health-professions university, reviewing as they do important health issues and reporting findings to the scientific and lay communities.

Obesity is a complicated problem, with ramifications which both scientists and members of the public at large can appreciate. Efforts to understand it more thoroughly and eventually to conquer it promise direct improvement in the quality of more lives than most scientific inquiries are likely to produce. It is a source of pride to the University that, under the leadership of Drs. Hadley Conn and Peter Kuo, chiefs of the UMD-RMS Department of Medicine and Division of Cardiology respectively, this learned gathering in pursuit of this most worthy end was convened and this volume achieved.

Stanley S. Bergen, Jr., M.D.
President, University of
Medicine and Dentistry of
New Jersey—Rutgers
Medical School

Foreword

The current federal administration has chosen to emphasize prevention as a major theme of its health programs. Cynics may say that the reason for this is that it is cheaper to promote health and prevent illness than to treat disease. Perhaps it is. Certainly, this volume on health and obesity focuses on one of the major preventable factors of disease in our society. There is even a significant literary and historical legacy describing the unfavorable relationship between health and obesity. Dickens' portrayal of Fat Joe in *The Pickwick Papers* and the decrease in mortality rates among residents of occupied countries in Europe during World War II, which was associated with reduction of food supplies and subsequent weight loss, are two of many examples of this relationship.

The Editors are to be commended for assembling this group of contributors who are outstanding investigators of obesity. These scientists have provided us with an invaluable update in understanding the science of obesity, its management, and its impact on health.

Richard C. Reynolds, M.D.
Dean, University of Medicine and Dentistry
of New Jersey—Rutgers Medical School

Preface

Numerous epidemiologic, metabolic, and cardiopulmonary studies have identified obesity as one of the common public health problems plaguing peoples of the affluent society. It predisposes the individual to a variety of chronic, degenerative diseases such as hypertension, hyperlipoproteinemia, cardiopulmonary diseases, diabetes mellitus, and others. This volume provides a comprehensive review of the current understanding of the complex interacting causative factors in obesity. Some of the disciplines involved range widely from physiology, biochemistry, neuropsychiatry, calorie, and nutrition. Based on the diverse pathophysiologic mechanisms of obesity a variety of management techniques including diet, exercise, behavior modification, pharmacologic therapy, and surgical procedures are used to control obesity with variable degrees of success.

This volume begins with a comprehensive overview of health and obesity. Epidemiologic studies reveal a large proportion of overweight subjects in the United States population. Early prevention of obesity to reduce the incidence of coronary heart disease, heart failure, and stroke is emphasized and discussed in detail.

Chapters that follow discuss the biochemistry and physiology of adipose tissue growth in man. A special effort is made to explain the biochemical, physiological, thermogenie, and anatomical differences between white and brown adipose tissues. Evidence to date indicates that although brown adipose tissue plays a role in the thermogenesis in human neonates, its role in the adult man is unclear. The complex determinants of human body fat content such as age, genetic influence, level of physical activity, diet palatability, variety of available food and the efficiency with which food energy is utilized are reviewed.

The major components of the regulatory system of body fat store such as the central nervous system, the specific neural pathways of feeding and satiety, and the neural link between ventromedial hypothalamus and brown adipose tissue are defined. A subset of mildly-to-moderately overweight patients who gain weight after adulthood with development of carbohydrate intolerance, hyperinsulinemia, exaggerated insulin response to carbohydrate feeding, hypertriglyceridemia (very-low-density lipoproteinemia elevation), depressed high-density-lipoprotein level, and mild hypertension are discussed. These patients are particularly prone to atherosclerosis. Data are presented to indicate the modulating roles of adrenergic receptors in the medial and lateral hypothalamus and peripheral signals on the feeding characteristics. Approaches to help obese patients such as the control of dietary energy intake, modification in the eating pattern, short-term use of liquid protein diet, and total fast are used according to specific indications. A comprehensive discussion presents evidence that behavior therapy is more effective than a variety of alternative treatments for mild and moderate obesity. At that time a detailed practical behavior modification program for obese subjects is provided.

The ineffectiveness of a conventional low calorie diet for massively obese patients is reemphasized. By using a two phase program, it has been found that a modified fast regimen can be an effective approach to weight control. The program is reinforced by the modification of eating habits, nutritional education, exercise, and frequent follow-up visits. The possible causes for confusion about the inappropriate clinical use of anorectic drugs for weight control in the treatment of obesity are enumerated. Innovation of combined anoretic drug therapy to reduce toxicity and maximize effectiveness is presented.

The volume concludes with a discussion of the three basic surgical procedures: the jejunoileal bypass, the gastric bypass, and gastroplasty for the treatment of grotesque patients. Surgical procedure(s) is supplemented with caloric control, behavior modification, and exercise to obtain long-term control of morbid obesity.

The editors believe that this volume accomplishes its aims in bringing the complex interacting factors of health and the menacing overweight problem into better focus, to direct and stimulate future research, and to apply and improve tthe current methods of treatment. This volume will be of interest to all physicians, surgeons, and researchers interested in the management of obese patients and in understanding underlying causal factors and physiological concomitants of obesity.

The Editors

Acknowledgments

We are grateful to Dr. Stanley S. Bergen, President, and Dr. Richard C. Reynolds, Dean, University of Medicine and Dentistry of New Jersey–Rutgers Medical School for their support, participation, and contributions to the symposium on which this volume is based.

We wish to give our heartiest thanks to Dr. G. Robert Moutrie, Assistant Vice-President and Director of Continuing Education and his hard-working staff, to Ms. Pat Reid and Ms. Lynn Grewe for their invaluable help, and to Mrs. Harriet Durmaskin for her able secretarial help.

We acknowledge Sandoz, Inc. for its generous support and the American Heart Association, Hunterdon-Somerset Heart Chapter for acting as cosponsor.

Contents

Contributors

Stanley S. Bergen, Jr., M.D. *University of Medicine and Dentistry of New Jersey, Rutgers Medical School, Piscataway, New Jersey 08854*

Elliot M. Berry, M.D., MRCP. *Laboratory of Human Behavior and Metabolism, Rockefeller University, New York, New York 10021*

George L. Blackburn, M.D., Ph.D. *Department of Surgery, Harvard Medical School, Cancer Research Institute, New England Deaconess Hospital, Boston, Massachusetts 02215*

George A. Bray, M.D. *Department of Medicine, University of Southern California School of Medicine, Los Angeles, California 90033*

Hadley L. Conn, Jr., M.D. *Department of Medicine, University of Medicine and Dentistry of New Jersey, Rutgers Medical School, Piscataway, New Jersey 08854*

Eugene A. DeFelice, M.D. *Department of Medicine, University of Medicine and Dentistry of New Jersey, Rutgers Medical School, Piscataway, New Jersey 08854*

Jules Hirsch, M.D. *Laboratory of Human Behavior and Metabolism, Rockefeller University, New York, New York 10021*

William B. Kannel, M.D. *Department of Medicine, Boston University School of Medicine, Boston, Massachusetts 02118*

Peter T. Kuo, M.D. *Department of Medicine, Division of Cardiovascular Diseases, University of Medicine and Dentistry of New Jersey, Rutgers Medical School, Piscataway, New Jersey 08854*

Louis Lasagna, M.D. *Departments of Pharmacology and Medicine, University of Rochester School of Medicine and Dentistry, Rochester, New York 14642*

Rudolph L. Leibel, M.D. *Laboratory of Human Behavior and Metabolism, Rockefeller University, New York, New York 10021*

Marijean M. Miller, B.A.*Nutrition Support Service, Cancer Research Institute, New England Deaconess Hospital, Boston, Massachusetts 02215*

Richard C. Reynolds, M.D. *Department of Medicine, University of Medicine and Dentistry of New Jersey, Rutgers Medical School, Piscataway, New Jersey 08854*

Albert J. Stunkard, M.D. *Department of Psychiatry, University of Pennsylvania School of Medicine, Philadelphia, Pennsylvania 19104*

Theodore B. Van Itallie, M.D. *St. Luke's Medical Service, St. Luke's-Roosevelt Hospital Center and Department of Medicine and Institute of Human Nutrition, Columbia University, College of Physicians and Surgeons, New York, New York 10025*

Victor Vertes, M.D. *Department of Medicine, Mount Sinai Medical Center, Cleveland, Ohio 44106*

Thomas A. Wadden, Ph.D. *Department of Psychiatry, University of Pennsylvania School of Medicine, Philadelphia, Pennsylvania 19104*

Health and Obesity, edited by H. L. Conn, Jr.,
E. A. DeFelice, and P. Kuo. Raven Press,
New York © 1983.

Health and Obesity: An Overview

William B. Kannel

*Department of Medicine, Boston University School of Medicine,
Boston, Massachusetts 02118*

The relationship of overweight to health is well documented but poorly understood. A variety of diseases occur in the obese in excess of the expected rate including: hypertension, hyperlipidemia, diabetes, gout, cardiovascular disease, gallbladder disease, and menstrual and ovarian irregularities. Most agree that obesity is hazardous to health and detrimental to well-being and, because of its multiple biological concomitants, its promotion of atherogenic traits, and its high prevalence, obesity constitutes a major public health problem.

However, despite the presumption that obesity is unhealthy and much research into its physiology, the determinants and health consequences of obesity remain controversial. Some investigators remain skeptical about some of the medical hazards despite extensive actuarial and epidemiologic evidence (29,33). Nevertheless, there is justified concern about the large number of overweight Americans (1). Because of the epidemic proportions of the problem, epidemiologic studies have been undertaken in an effort to gain insights into its determinants. Long-term prospective studies have been implemented to examine the health consequences, risks, and disadvantages of obesity, usually as a part of a more comprehensive study of cardiovascular risk factors (20). These provide the best insights.

INDICES

Obesity is best defined as a surplus of body fat. Accurate determination of body fat composition, although technologically feasible, requires procedures that are not applicable for clinical medical practice or epidemiologic investigation (13). Most studies of adiposity have been based on crude approximations of body fat composition from height, weight, girth, and skinfold thickness measurements.

Although there are various ways of translating height and weight measurements into estimates of adiposity, they all tend to be highly correlated (20). There is little reason to believe that any particular index is actually superior in providing a precise estimate of the proportion of body weight contained in adipose tissue.

The adipose tissue mass is the product of the number and size of adipocytes. Hyperplasia occurs *in utero*, during the first year of life, at puberty, and probably also when adipocytes achieve maximum cell size. In all forms of obesity, adipocytes

1

hypertrophied by their fat content are the rule. It has been suggested that only the hypertrophic obesity of adult onset is in theory reversible (13). It has been noted that obesity may be generalized or central (truncal) in distribution with the hypertrophic variety more generalized. Somatotypists insist that endomorphy is somehow distinct from obesity. Little information on the specific biologic accompaniments or disease potential of these varieties of obesity is available.

Fat cell mass is not well correlated with fat cell size and when increased generally implies an increased cell number. Since fat cells are reported to reach their adult number by age 18, increased body fat acquired in adulthood is believed to result primarily from increased fat cell size.

As regards ideal or optimal weight, the appropriate standard of comparison is elusive (7,8). In environments characterized by a harsh climate and intermittent food supply, obesity may actually enhance survival. Associated hazards to health and life expectancy are important considerations, but these may vary in different cultures. There are also genetic considerations. The psychosocial consequences are important considerations in Western cultures.

The proportion of body fat generally accepted as "normal" is 15 to 20% for men and 20 to 25% for women although these usual values are not necessarily optimal. A 10 to 20% excess of body fat over these usual values is generally considered "obesity."

Of the different methods for quantifying body fat, measurement of skinfold thickness appears to be the most practical alternative and more specific than the more precisely determined relative weight. However, there is little agreement on how much body fat is optimal by any of these measures.

PREVALENCE

By any definition, obesity is highly prevalent in the United States (Table 1). Despite powerful psychosocial forces of fashion, youth cultism, and health concern, weights tend to creep inexorably upward with age in both sexes until late in life (36). This may be largely a cohort difference reflecting the fact that men born later in this century are consistently heavier than those the same age born earlier. However, longitudinal data of relative weights and skinfolds in the Framingham Study indicate that both men and women get fatter until late in life when they tend to lose weight (20).

Although there are large differences in weight and weights tend to rise with age to middle age, weight is nevertheless under sensitive biologic control. Despite wide short-term fluctuation, weights are highly characteristic of persons and even 18 years apart correlate at 0.75 (20). In general, obesity is an insidious disorder resulting from almost imperceptible weight increments.

Overweight, using common definitions, is as prevalent as any of the major cardiovascular risk factors excepting the cigarette habit. Most data on the incidence and prevalence of obesity involve surveys employing body weight measurements in relation to height and age. Current estimates of the prevalence of obesity are

TABLE 1. *Prevalence of overweight—percent of population deviating by 20% or more from desirable weight[a]*

	Men		Women	
Age	1960–62	1971–74	1960–62	1971–74
20–74	14.5	14.0	25.1	23.8
20–24	9.6	7.4	9.1	9.6
25–34	13.3	13.6	14.8	17.1
35–44	14.9	17.0	23.2	24.3
45–54	16.7	15.8	28.9	27.8
55–64	15.8	15.1	38.6	34.7
65–74	14.6	13.4	38.8	31.5

[a]Estimated from regression equation of weight on height for men and women ages 20–29 years, obtained from HANES I. United States, Health Examination Survey 1960–62 and Health and Nutrition Examination Survey 1971–74. See ref. 1a.

variable, but all indicate a high rate of occurrence in Western affluent society (Table 1). There is also evidence that its prevalence is increasing (36). There is also some geographic variation in prevalence within the United States.

The prevalence of obesity, which is found at all ages, increases with age at least under middle age. The apparent decline thereafter must be interpreted recognizing the decrease in lean body mass with advanced age. It is unlikely that the increase in prevalence of obesity with age is an inevitable consequence of aging or genetic makeup.

An epidemic of obesity continues in most subgroups of the United States. A greater proportion of women than men are obese and black women are more likely to be obese than white women. Among adults with incomes below the poverty level the women, but not the men, tend to become more obese (50).

If the insurance criteria of optimal weight are applied to the National Health Examination Survey data for 1960–1962, almost 30% of the men and women are 20% above *optimal* weight. The average Framingham subject was approximately 20% above optimal weight and more than 15% of the men and 20% of the women had relative weights at least 30% above optimum. As many as 3% of the men and 9% of the women were massively obese (i.e., 50% above optimum).

DETERMINANTS

There is wide agreement that obesity results from an intake of calories in excess of energy expended. Most obesity is a chronic, resistant condition of excessive fat tissue in the absence of obvious genetic or hormonal disorders. Although it is true that overeating is fundamental to the problem, there are genetic and environmental factors that affect how food is metabolized. Persons fed the same diet do have different lipid values and blood sugars and may well also respond differently in the amount of energy stored as fat.

Despite the presumption that obesity is unhealthy and a large body of research into its physiology, there has been little progress in unraveling its psychosocial, metabolic, and genetic determinants. Once obesity is sustained, the evidence suggests that it tends to become self-perpetuating as if homeostatic mechanisms have been reset to maintain a heavier weight. Whether this is a consequence of permanent hyperplasia of insulin-insensitive fat cells, a blunted ability to regulate caloric intake to need, or psychosocial factors, is unclear (33).

Although it is universally agreed that obesity reflects an excess of caloric intake over expenditure of energy, the psychosocial and metabolic determinants of obesity are poorly understood. It is likely that there are multiple causes of obesity.

There is some evidence that adaptive changes in thermogenesis accompany changes in diet. Undernutrition is generally associated with a decreased metabolic rate and more efficient utilization and storage of calories whereas overfeeding increases the metabolic rate and dissipation of calories as heat (30). Diet-induced alterations in sympathetic activity may be responsible for these adaptive changes in thermogenesis mediated through insulin, which may have important implications for the development of obesity and its promotion of cardiovascular disease. There is a need for more research into the burning of calories and appetite regulation (30).

Adipose tissue cellularity is believed to be fundamental to the problem of intractable obesity. Enlargement of the adipose tissue depot occurs either by increase in adipocyte size or number or both. In general, the earlier in life obesity is established and the more severe it becomes, the more likely there is hypercellularity. Although hypercellularity can also occur in adult life and in those not massively obese, once established it seems to be irreversible. Hypercellularity is most likely to occur within the first 2 years of life or around puberty. In obese children there is often a marked expansion of the adipose tissue depot throughout childhood involving both cellular enlargement and proliferation. When maximum cell size is reached, adipocyte cell division appears to be stimulated.

Weight loss and reduction in adipose tissue mass is accompanied by a change in cell size alone with the number remaining constant despite massive weight loss. This may explain why long-standing, severe obesity is so intractable.

The adipose cell hypothesis postulates that adipocyte proliferation is excessively stimulated in the last trimester of pregnancy, early infancy, or adolescence causing irreversible hypercellular expansion of adipose tissue that may play a role in perpetuation of one type of obesity. The mechanisms by which adipose hypercellularity or hypertrophy might perpetuate the obese state remain speculative. Feedback mechanisms mediated through adipose cell number and size have been postulated.

Whereas it is undoubtedly true that obesity derives from an excessive intake of calories over energy expenditure, the reasons for continued overindulgence and the refractory nature of the condition seem complex. Genetic, metabolic, endocrine, and nutritional influences are probably all involved. However, the evolution of obesity is strongly influenced by social, economic, racial, and ethnic factors (8,17).

Obese parents tend to generate obese children and obese children tend to become obese adults (2,11). Approximately 80% of obese children were found to become obese adults and one-half of massively obese adults were found to have been obese infants. Nevertheless, the extent to which obesity in infancy and childhood is an important reservoir of adult obesity needs further clarification. Siblings tend to share obesity but this also applies to adopted children (18).

The trend to lifetime obesity is more pronounced in women than men. Long-standing obesity, once established, is often intractable, suggesting a self-perpetuating phenomenon. Black women are at greater risk than white women whereas white men are apt to be more obese than black men. These racial differences tend to disappear in subjects of the same socioeconomic status. Pregnancy is also a common precursor of obesity and obese women tend to reproduce at a faster pace.

Obesity has been reported to be associated with a variety of psychological problems (24). However, it is not clear how much is cause and how much effect. The majority of obese persons seem no more prone to emotional disturbances than lean persons. The emotional burden of being fat in a society that lauds leanness and stigmatizes obesity is considerable although not precisely quantified.

It has been suggested that the obese are less able to perceive internal feeding cues and respond more to the sight of food. Like man, adult laboratory animals when supplied highly palatable food *ad libitum* tend to overeat and become obese and hyperinsulinemic. This is reversible on return to conventional food. The incidence of obesity is highest in populations whose diet is high in fat and where physical activity is low.

The fact that there are secular trends in weight in genetically similar persons, such as the offspring of the Framingham cohort, suggests environmental influences. The offspring males were found to be distinctly heavier than their parents were at the same age 20 years previously; whereas the females were lighter. Nonphysiologic factors play a major role in determining energy intake and expenditure. Culturally determined and socially reinforced attitudes are undoubtedly important. However, intentional self-regulation appears to be fragile, and conscious dietary restraint easily disrupted by a multitude of influences that induce overeating (22).

Both environmental and genetic factors must be accorded major roles in obesity. Pronounced secular trends and social strata differences suggest an important role for life-style. However, there is much to suggest a genetic predisposition to obesity from experience in animal husbandry, twins raised apart, the correlations of weights of parents with natural versus adopted children, strains of rodents with genetically transmitted obesity, and familial aggregation of obesity.

Obesity definitely tends to run in families, but not necessarily because of genetic influences. The fact that spouses as well as siblings tend to share obesity suggests an obesity-promoting home environment. However, since there is little tendency for spouse aggregation of obesity to increase with the duration of marriage, assortive mating may be involved.

SOCIAL FACTORS

Striking associations between the prevalence of obesity and socioeconomic status have been reported, particularly in women (19). Social mobility was also found to be related to obesity with those moving upward least obese and those moving downward in social status most obese (19). Also successive generations of families in the United States were shown to be less obese than those who went before. Religious affiliation has also been connected with obesity with Jews most obese and Episcopalians least obese (50). These findings have also been noted in the English culture (43). In a Western urban setting social factors have more influence on the weight of women than men. The inverse relationship between obesity and socioeconomic status has been found to be well established as early as adolescence (23,51,53).

In less affluent societies an increasing standard of living is associated with a *greater* prevalence of obesity (16). In a society with a surfeit of good food and drink and shrinking opportunities for exercise as an obligatory condition of daily life, obesity would seem inevitable, particularly when dining is viewed as a form of entertainment.

MORTALITY

Investigations of the mortality experience of insured lives since the turn of the century have consistently indicated an association of overweight with excess mortality (3,31,44). The excess mortality associated with obesity is in general greater in men than women, except possibly for the massively obese where the two sexes seem to have a similar mortality (Table 2).

The actuarial experience of United States insurance companies in the past indicated a direct relationship between overweight and mortality such that the less the weight the lower the risk of death to a point of minimum mortality well below average weight for height (44). More recent experience indicates a change so that optimal weight now is at a more plump level, and more lean weights (20% below average) appear to be associated with an excess mortality (Table 2).

The findings of the Framingham Study did not accord with the earlier insurance experience. In this unselected population sample minimum mortality occurred around the average (slightly plump) weight with increased mortality for those weighing either more or less than average (Fig. 1). The apparent excess mortality in underweight persons in both the recent insurance and Framingham experience is not well understood. In the Framingham Study this excess mortality in underweight persons persists even if those with known cancer, diabetes, or cardiovascular disease are excluded from the analysis (45). The higher proportion of lean persons who survive could be a confounding factor. Approximately 80% of men in the leanest weight category were found to be cigarette smokers, compared to less than one-half the obese subjects. Hence a substantial part of the excess mortality in lean persons is attributable to the large number of cigarette smokers. Lean cigarette smokers experienced a mortality often higher than all but the most overweight cigarette smokers. Most of this excess mortality in the lean cigarette smokers was from noncardiovascular causes. At any weight, the cigarette smoker has a higher mortality than the nonsmoker (Fig. 2). However, the higher proportion of lean persons who

TABLE 2. *Mortality experience in relation to deviation from average weight*

Sex	Deviation from average weight (%)	Insured lives		General population 1959–1972[c]
		1954–1972[a] (provisional)	1935–1954[b]	
Men	−20	105	90	110
	−10	94	95	100
	+10	111	113	107
	+20	120	125	121
	+30	133	142	137
	+40	150	167	162
	+50	171	200	210
	+60	195	260	—
Women	−20	110	99	100
	−10	97	95	95
	+10	106	109	108
	+20	110	121	123
	+30	125	130	138
	+40	136	—	162
	+50	150	—	200
	+60	—	—	—

[a]Society of Actuaries and Association Life Insurance Medical Directors, Build and Blood Pressure Study, 1979.
[b]Society of Actuaries and Association Life Insurance Medical Directors, Build and Blood Pressure Study, 1959.
[c]American Cancer Society, Cancer Prevention Study.

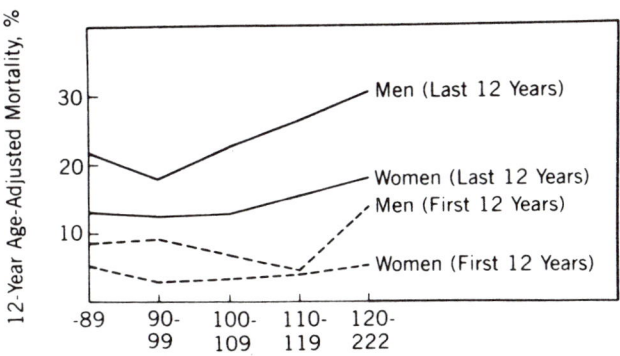

FIG. 1. Mortality in first 12 years and in last 12 years of study by Framingham relative weight measured at exam 1. Men and women, 30–59 at entry excluding those with disease: Framingham study: 24 year follow-up.

smoke did not appear to account entirely for the excess mortality in the leannest group. The shape of the mortality curve in relation to weight is similar in smokers and nonsmokers in the Framingham Study. However, there was a paucity of data in the nonsmoking lean group.

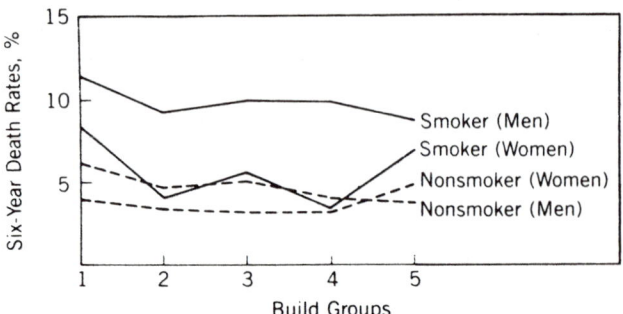

FIG. 2. Six-year age-adjusted death rates by body build and smoking status.

The latest data on mortality raise questions about standards of ideal or optimal weight for the American population. How lean is it desirable for the average American to become? Also, considering the rather striking relationship of obesity to potentially lethal conditions such as coronary disease, gallbladder disease, diabetes, and hypertension, the mortality risk gradients associated with obesity are surprisingly modest.

The excess mortality in lean persons requires further study. Overt illness did not account for this in the Framingham Study. However, the study did confirm the clinical impression that persons who lose weight without deliberately dieting do indeed have a higher mortality rate (18,45). The caloric intake of men who died was found to be lower, reflecting loss of appetite. The fact that mortality in the Framingham cohort showed a greater tendency to increase with relative weight later than in the first 12 years suggests that low weight reflects subclinical disease.

There is some indication that mortality trends in relation to weight may change over time. Early this century there was a distinct excess mortality at below average weights. This later disappeared and now the 1979 Body Build and Blood Pressure Study again shows a distinctly higher mortality at weights 20% below average (45). The earlier experience was chiefly accounted for by tuberculosis, which causes relatively few deaths today. Any mortality experience includes some persons with unrecognized illness whose weights are affected by the underlying process. This renders the procedure of establishing an ideal weight on the basis of prospective experience suspect.

The data on hand raise questions about the benefits of weight reduction in persons of average weight. However, both the Framingham Study and the insurance studies show that it is worse to be obese than lean, particularly as regards propensity to cardiovascular mortality. Those 15% or more underweight in the Framingham Study died sooner, but their deaths could not be traced to a single cause such as cancer. The increased mortality could be demonstrated in relation to being underweight even after 12 years had elapsed, tending to eliminate the possibility of cancer as the cause of both the underweight and excess mortality. In the insurance studies their men died of pneumonia, suicide, digestive tract diseases, cancer, and hypertension. Their women died of suicide, digestive disease, pneumonia, and stroke.

MEDICAL CONSEQUENCES

Many medical conditions have been found to be associated with obesity, including cardiovascular disease, gallbladder disease, menstrual irregularities, diabetes, and gout. Although the pathogenetic mechanisms are often obscure, the association is quite clear, and, because correction of the obesity often improves the associated disease process, a causal relationship seems likely.

Menstrual, Uterine, and Ovarian Abnormalities

There is a substantial body of data linking obesity to prolonged menstrual cycles, menorrhagia, irregular menses, and excess facial hair in women (21). Ovarian pathology has been found to occur in excess in women with morbid obesity (14). Obesity promotes anovulatory cycles and polycystic ovaries. This has been attributed to prolonged estrogen stimulation.

In 14 of 15 investigations, obesity has been linked to endometrial carcinoma (5). Teenage obesity has been found to be associated with a 1.6-fold increased risk of endometrial carcinoma compared to lean teenagers. Excessive estrogen stimulation leading to cystic glandular hyperplasia may be responsible.

Although obesity has been incriminated as a risk factor for breast and endometrial cancer, there is no evidence from trials to indicate whether weight reduction can protect against these neoplasms. Increased estrogens in obese women, associated with anovulatory cycles, subject their endometrial tissues to excessive unopposed estrogen stimulation. Anovulatory menstrual cycles and luteal failure also have been shown to be risk factors for breast cancer.

Cardiovascular Hazards

There is consistent and substantial evidence connecting obesity with an increased risk of cardiovascular disease deriving from case studies and prospective population studies. The relationship between relative weight and severity of atherosclerosis per se is less clear. Postmortem surveys have generally failed to show a clear relationship between obesity and atherosclerosis. This may derive from assessments of weights during the chronic terminal illness.

Prospective studies have uniformly shown a relationship of obesity to cardiovascular disease but not always an independent effect. In general, long-term studies have shown more substantial relationships. There is some evidence to suggest that obesity acquired between ages 20 to 40 years may have a greater impact than that which occurs after age 40 (39). Morbid obesity is associated with serious cardiorespiratory illness (25). Lesser degrees of overweight are variably associated with excess morbidity. In the Pooling Project mild to moderate overweight was accompanied by an increased risk of coronary heart disease (CHD), again, only under age 50 (38).

In the Framingham Study there was a distinct excess incidence of cardiovascular disease and death in persons who were overweight, the excess over expected increasing with the degree of overweight (20,27,42). To a considerable extent this is attributable to the fact that as people gain weight their blood pressure, blood lipids, and glucose values tend to rise; the effect is less in women than men (4). Although the association of obesity with cardiovascular risk factors is weaker in women than men, obesity itself is at least as strongly associated with cardiovascular disease in women as in men (28,42). Consistent with observations elsewhere, the strength of the association of obesity with cardiovascular disease incidence wanes with advancing age and beyond age 65 the association is no longer statistically significant for any cardiovascular disease endpoint (42).

From multivariate analysis it is evident that much of the effect of obesity is mediated through associated cardiovascular risk factors. However, the obese have a doubled risk of brain infarction and cardiac failure and a distinct, but more modest, excess risk of CHD. Intermittent claudication is an anomaly, which, in the Framingham cohort, was more likely to occur in lean than obese persons (Fig. 3).

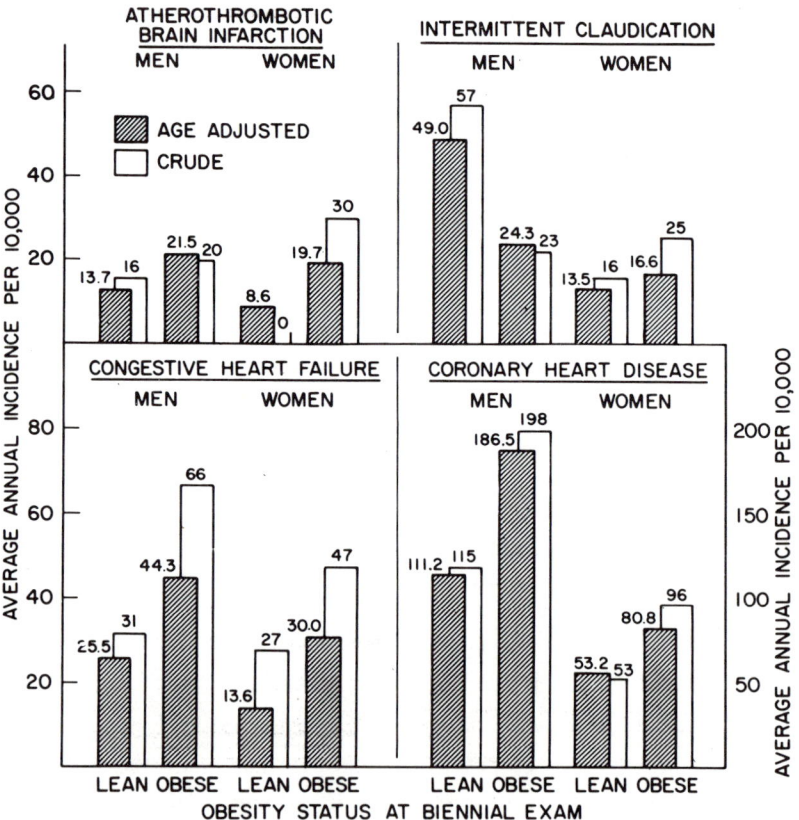

FIG. 3. Risk of cardiovascular disease according to obesity status; men and women, ages 45–74 at exam: Framingham Study: 18 year follow-up.

Gallbladder Disease

Autopsy data, case reports, and prospective population studies have all shown a strong relationship between obesity and gallbladder disease. There is much evidence relating gallbladder disease to obesity at all ages and this persists in women, even adjusting for parity (41). Obese persons tend to hypersecrete biliary cholesterol, which is more lithogenic, being disproportionately saturated with cholesterol relative to bile salts and phospholipids.

Arthritis

An association between arthritis and obesity has been claimed. A study of women has shown a 55% greater occurrence of arthritis in those who were more than 85% above desirable weight compared to those who were less than 10% overweight (40). It is frequently observed in clinical practice that weight loss often reduces symptoms of bone and joint disease, especially that involving weight-bearing joints.

Osteoarthritis of the knees and hips is probably a greater cause of disability in the obese than is recognized. However, evidence linking the two is based almost exclusively on clinical impressions and case reports. Population-based prevalence information and estimates of the actual risk entailed are not possible.

Psychosocial Disability

Studies of selected samples have shown that various kinds of psychosocial disability are more common among the obese. The obese are subject to social, economic, and other discrimination (10,32). It is clear that in the contemporary American middle class obesity is a social stigma. Possibly as a consequence, the obese are subject to self disparagement and have a poor self-image. However, there are few representative large-scale population studies from which to draw firm conclusions and even fewer clinical trials assessing changes in psychosocial features. However, studies of psychosocial function in severely obese subjects following intestinal bypass surgery have indicated improvement.

Surgical and Anesthetic Risks

Obese persons undergoing surgery more often encounter anesthetic, diagnostic, surgical, and postoperative problems. Postoperative complications include hematomas, wound infections, incision dehiscence, pulmonary atelectasis, and thromboembolic complications (49).

Biological Concomitants

Although overt abnormalities severe enough to be labeled disease are uncommon, obesity does produce a modest change in blood pressure, blood lipids, glucose tolerance, and uric acid values. Changes in blood volume, cardiac output, and pulmonary function have been noted with massive obesity.

Blood Pressure

There is a well-established relationship between overweight and blood pressure elevation (6,12,15,46–48,52). Intervention trials have suggested that weight reduction is accompanied by a corresponding reduction in blood pressure independent of salt intake (50). Spontaneous weight fluctuations in the Framingham Study were found to be associated with corresponding changes in blood pressure. Because there is also a subsequent rise in blood pressure with regained weight, a causal relationship is likely. Since blood pressure is altered in relation to changes in body weight, body fat rather than some other feature of increased body mass appears to be the culprit. Positive correlations have been shown to exist between blood pressure and various indices of adiposity (12,27,47,52). Recent studies have shown that all components of blood pressure are related to percent body fat, total body fat mass, and fat cell number. Significant correlations with lean body mass or fat cell size are less well established. These findings have now been extended to children where various measures of body fatness have been shown to be related to blood pressure.

Change in relative weight was the most potent factor found to be associated with longitudinal trends in blood pressure in the Framingham cohort (Fig. 4). One standard deviation in weight change was associated with a 6.5 mm Hg change in blood pressure in 10 years (4). This relationship is not a fat-arm artifact since it can be demonstrated from forearm blood pressures and even intraarterial pressures.

Although adiposity is not the chief determinant of hypertension, the association has been demonstrated in multiple cultures and in the young as well as in adults. This well-established relationship of adiposity to blood pressure is of uncertain pathogenesis. Obesity has been found to be associated with enhanced sympathetic nervous activity, which could account for the blood pressure elevation (30). The intravascular volume is expanded in the obese, accompanied by an increased stroke volume and cardiac output and this may play a role. Obese subjects also excrete increased quantities of salt irrespective of plasma renin activity (35), perhaps in response to mobilization of natriuretic hormone by the expanded blood volume (34). However, more research is clearly needed. It has also been alleged that truncal fat is more closely correlated with blood pressure than limb fat, but this requires confirmation (5).

Blood Lipids

Development of obesity affects the various blood lipids. In the Framingham cohort, changes in weight were found to be mirrored by changes in serum total cholesterol (Figs. 4, 5). However, other lipids and lipoproteins are more profoundly influenced by weight gain.

Some lipid and lipoprotein accompaniments of obesity and its association with glucose intolerance were examined over 18 years of follow-up in the Framingham cohort. Whereas low-density lipoproteins (LDL) and very-low density lipoproteins (VLDL) were positively correlated with relative weight, high-density lipoprotein (HDL) cholesterol was inversely correlated. (28). The association was strongest for

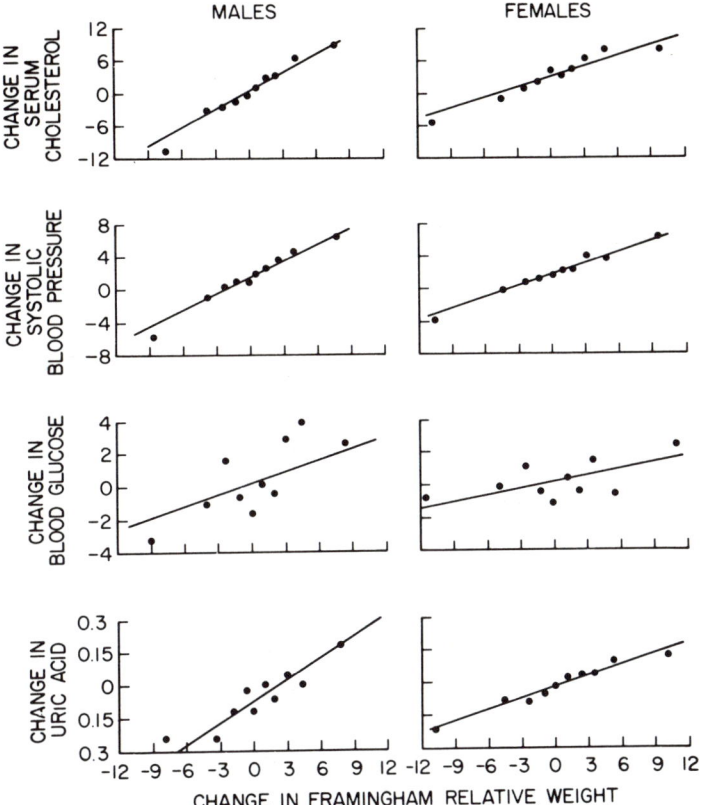

FIG. 4. Changes in characteristic values with change in Framingham relative weight.

HDL, varying little by age and sex. Triglycerides were a close second, and were more closely associated with obesity in men than women and in younger than older persons.

In general, degree of overweight was more closely related to blood lipids in men than women of the same age. Also, the strength of the association was generally greater in younger than older persons. Since all the lipids promoted by obesity are cardiovascular risk factors, it would appear that obesity is atherogenic. In particular, it has been shown that the ratio of LDL/HDL or total cholesterol/HDL is adversely affected (Fig. 5). This lipid profile has been shown to be the best single predictor of CHD (26).

Diabetes and Glucose Intolerance

Health surveys have convincingly shown that obesity is an important predisposing factor for glucose intolerance or diabetes (Fig. 6). However, prospective studies following subjects for the onset of diabetes or glucose intolerance are sparse and often restricted to specific ethnic and racial groups (2). Nevertheless, the degree

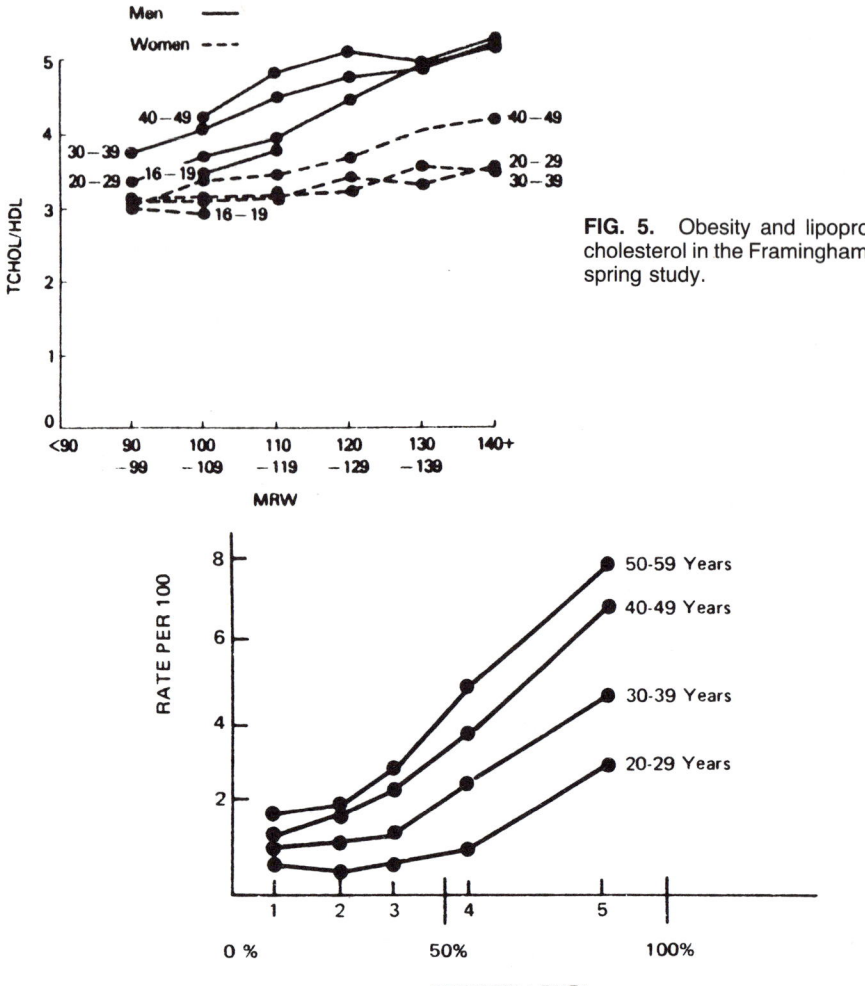

FIG. 5. Obesity and lipoprotein cholesterol in the Framingham offspring study.

FIG. 6. Obesity and age-specific occurrence rates for women with a history of adult-onset diabetes.

and duration of obesity is the factor most strongly related to adult-onset diabetes in the United States (37).

In the Framingham Study a cohort of 5,082 men and women aged 33 to 67 were followed prospectively for 14 years for the occurrence of glucose intolerance in order to determine what factors predisposed. Using multivariate analysis, it was found that in either sex future glucose intolerance was highly associated with casual blood glucose values (within the normal range), VLDL, and relative weight (Table 3). Both obesity and lipoprotein abnormalities were shown to be independent predictors of subsequent glucose intolerance. In women, particularly, obesity influenced the risk of developing glucose intolerance more than any other factor, including

TABLE 3. *Standardized multivariate logistic regression coefficients predicting glucose intolerance over 14 years: The Framingham Study*

Characteristic	Men (coefficient)	Women (coefficient)
Age	0.16	−0.11
Metropolitan relative weight	0.38[a]	0.48[a]
Claudication	0.17[b]	0.08
Uric acid	−0.06	0.18
LDL	−0.18	−0.03
VLDL	0.22[b]	0.27[b]
Hemoglobin	0.07	0.34[b]
Systolic blood pressure	−0.03	0.16
Glucose	0.50[a]	0.33[a]

[a]$p < 0.001$ and [b]$p < 0.01$, using two-tailed Student's t-test.

prior blood glucose. Women in the top 20% of weight distribution represented 48% of the total number of women developing glucose intolerance over 14 years in the Framingham cohort. Those in the upper quintile of relative weight developed 4 times as much glucose intolerance as those in the lower quintile. Weight alone was able to predict 45% of future glucose intolerance in women.

The precise nature of the relationship of obesity to impaired glucose intolerance is incompletely understood. Obesity somehow induces impaired carbohydrate metabolism and increased insulin secretion. Weight loss can correct this by reducing the hyperinsulinemia and restoring normal glucose tolerance, suggesting a causal or aggravating role. Weight changes in the Framingham Study were mirrored by corresponding changes in blood glucose (Fig. 4). The insulin resistance of obese persons appears to be responsible for the hyperglycemia of obesity but it is not clear whether this is a cell membrane receptor problem, or due to intracellular metabolic dysfunction. Also, the hyperinsulinemia in the obese is often unaccompanied by hyperglycemia. However, whatever the mechanism, obesity clearly impairs glucose metabolism and affects insulin secretion.

Gout

Gout has long been linked to overweight. In the Framingham Study both uric acid values and clinical gout have been shown to be associated with relative weight (Fig. 4). This relationship has also been shown for women (40). The connection between purine metabolism and adiposity is poorly understood. There is also longitudinal data relating change in weight to corresponding changes in uric acid values (4). This is consistent with the clinical impression that weight control tends to reduce the frequency of gouty attacks.

PREVENTIVE IMPLICATIONS

Despite many uncertainties about the determinants and hazards of obesity, the mechanism for its adverse biologic concomitants, and the efficacy of correcting it, obesity control looms large as possibly the chief hygenic means currently available for the control of major chronic and degenerative disease.

There is no other single measure that can simultaneously improve all of the atherogenic precursors of cardiovascular disease. Weight reduction has been shown to improve blood pressure, the total cholesterol/HDL ratio, and uric acid and glucose tolerance (Figs. 4, 5).

No better recommendation is available for the avoidance of gallbladder disease, diabetes, gout, or degenerative arthritis.

Obesity, like many other chronic disorders, is more often controllable than curable. A greater sense of urgency is needed since it is more likely to respond to management if corrected early rather than late in its course. Also, like most chronic diseases, exacerbations and remissions are commonplace. The earlier in life it is established and the more pronounced it is, the more resistant obesity is to treatment (9). Because it is likely to be intractable, gross obesity is better prevented than cured.

Compared to other risk factors, obesity ranks quite low in men, but somewhat higher in women, as a direct predisposing influence on cardiovascular morbidity and mortality. However, because it reversibly promotes powerful atherogenic traits such as hypertension, diabetes, and lipid aberrations, reduction of overweight is one of the most important hygenic measures available for the control of cardiovascular disease. Also, because few other measures are available, it is important in preventive programs for gallbladder disease, diabetes, gout, arthritis, and uterine disease.

For those who are skeptical that obesity poses a hazard to cardiovascular health, only a trial demonstrating that correction of long-standing obesity does in fact prolong life will suffice. Because of our inability to date to achieve and sustain control of such obesity, this evidence is going to be a long time in coming. Since weight control is logically the initial approach for correcting or avoiding hypertension, lipid disorders, and diabetes, we cannot afford to await indefinitely such elusive proofs of efficacy. Although there is no sound basis for predicting the benefits of rigorous weight control, it has been estimated from the Framingham Study data that if everyone were at optimal weight we would have 25% less CHD and 35% fewer events of cardiac failure and strokes (20). This potential benefit seems worthy of continuing to seek ways to better control or avoid obesity.

Although no prospective study is likely because of the notorious difficulty in persuading the obese to maintain an optimal weight, the effort to corroborate the estimated benefits of correcting obesity is justified by the rationale. Obesity could probably be prevented by inculcating more hygenic eating practices in early childhood, but ignorance, indifference, ingrained cultural patterns, and commercially-vested interests impose formidable barriers.

The unsatisfactory state of treatment of obesity is attested to by the perennial fad diets and continued high prevalence of the condition. The causes, prevention, and cure of obesity are probably the least well understood and most urgently in need of investigation of all the contributors to major cardiovascular and other chronic illnesses.

REFERENCES

1. Abraham, S., and Johnson, C. L. (1980): Prevalence of severe obesity in adults in the United States. *Am. J. Clin. Nutr.*, 33:364–369.
1a. Abraham, S., and Johnson, C. L. (19XX): Overweight adults 20–74 years of age: United States, 1971–74. National Center for Health Statistics. Advance Data No. 51, D.H.E.W. Hyattsville, Maryland.
2. Abraham, S., and Nordsieck, M. (1960): Relationship of excess weight of children and adults. *Public Health Rep.*, 75:263–273.
3. Armstrong, D. B., Dublin, L. I., Wheatley, G. M., and Marks, H. H. (1951): Obesity and its relation to health and disease. *JAMA*, 147:1007–1014.
4. Ashley, F. W., Jr., and Kannel, W. B. (1974): Relation of weight change to changes in atherogenic traits. The Framingham Study. *J. Chronic Dis.*, 27:103–114.
5. Blitzer, P. H., Blitzer, E. C., and Rimm, A. A. (1976): Association between teenage obesity and cancer in 56,111 women. *Prev. Med.*, 5:20–31.
6. Bøe, J., Humerfelt, S., and Wedervaag, F. (1957): The blood pressure in a population. Blood pressure readings and height and weight determinations in the adult population of the city of Bergen. *Acta Med. Scand.*, 157 (Suppl 321):1–336.
7. Bray, G. A. (1969): Definition, measurement and classification of the syndromes of obesity. *Int. J. Obes.*, 2:99–122.
8. Bray, G. A., editor (1976): *Fogarty International Center Series on Preventive Medicine, Vol. 2: Obesity in Perspective, Parts 1 and 2.* D.H.E.W. Publication No. (N.I.H.) 76–852.
9. Brook, C. G. D. (1974): Critical periods in childhood obesity. In: *Obesity*, edited by W. L. Burland, P. D. Samuel, and J. Yudkin, pp. 85–104. Churchill Livingstone, Edinburgh.
10. Cahnman, W. J. (1968): The stigma of obesity. *Sociol. Q.*, 9:283–299.
11. Charney, E., Goodman, H. C., and McBride, M. (1975): Childhood antecedents of adult obesity: Do chubby infants become obese adults? *N. Engl. J. Med.*, 295:6–9.
12. Chiang, B. N., Perluran, L. V., and Epstein, F. H. (1969): Overweight and hypertension: A review. *Circulation*, 39:403–421.
13. Durnin, J. V. G. A., and Womersley, J. (1974): Body fat assessed from total body density and its estimation from skinfold thickness: Measurements on 481 men and women aged from 16 to 72 years. *Br. J. Nutr.*, 32:77–97.
14. Fisher, E. R., Gregorio, R., Stephan, T., Nolan, S., and Danowski, T. S. (1974): Ovarian changes in women with morbid obesity. *Obstet. Gynecol.*, 44:839–844.
15. Florey, C., Due, V., and Acheson, R. (1969): Blood pressure as it relates to physique, blood glucose and serum cholesterol. In: *Vital and Health Statistics*. P.H.S. Publication No. 1000, Series 11, No. 34, pp. 1–29.
16. Garb, J. L., Garb, J. R., and Stunkard, A. J. (1975): Social factors and obesity in Navaho Indian children. In: *Recent Advances in Obesity Research*, pp. 37–39. Newman Publishing, London.
17. Garn, S. M. (1976): Trends in fatness and the origins of obesity. *Pediatrics*, 57:4.
18. Garn, S. M., Bailey, S. M., and Higgins, I. T. T. (1976): Fatness similarities in adopted pairs, a letter to the editor. *Am. J. Clin. Nutr.*, 29:1067.
18a. Garrison, R. J., Wilson, P. W., Castelli, W. P., Feinleib, M., Kannel, W. B., and McNamara, P. M. (1980): Obesity and lipoprotein cholesterol in the Framingham Offspring Study. *Metabolism*, 29:1053–1060.
19. Goldblatt, P. B., Moore, M. E., and Stunkard, A. J. (1965): Social factors in obesity. *JAMA*, 192:1039–1044.
20. Gordon, T., and Kannel, W. B. (1973): The effects of overweight on cardiovascular diseases. *Geriatrics*, 28:80–88.

21. Hartz, A., Wong, A., Katayama, K. P., and Rimm, A. A. (1979): The association of obesity with anovulatory cycles and related menstrual abnormalities in 36,081 women. *Int. J. Obes.*, 3:57–73.
22. Herman, C. P., and Mac, D. (1975): Restrained and unrestrained eating. *J. Pers.*, 43:647–660.
23. Heuneman, R. L. (1969): Factors associated with teenage obesity. In: *Obesity*, edited by N. L. Wilson, pp. 55–65. F.A. Davis Company, Philadelphia.
24. Jordon, H. A. (1976): Psychological factors associated with obesity. In: Bray 19(1):50–52.
25. Kaltman, A. J., and Goldring, R. M. (1976): Role of circulatory congestion in the cardiorespiratory failure of obesity. *Am. J. Med.*, 60:654–663.
26. Kannel, W. B., and Castelli, W. P. (1980): Prognostic implications of blood lipid measurements. In: *Prognosis*, edited by J. F. Fries and G. E. Ehrujat, pp. 263–268. Charles Press Publ. Maryland.
27. Kannel, W. B., and Gordon, T. (1979): Obesity and some physiological and medical concomitants. The Framingham Study. In: *Obesity in America*, edited by G. A. Bray, pp. 125–163. N.I.H. Publication No. 79–359.
28. Kannel, W. B., Gordon, T., and Castelli, W. P. (1979): Obesity, lipids and glucose tolerance: The Framingham Study. *Am. J. Clin. Nutr.*, 32:1238–1245.
29. Keys, A., Aravanis, C., Blackburn, H., VanBuckem, F.S.P., Busina, R., Djordevic, B. S., Findanza, F. F., Karvonen, M. J., Menotti, A., Puddu, V., and Taylor, H. L. (1972): Coronary heart disease: Overweight and obesity as risk factors. *Ann. Intern. Med.*, 77:15–27.
30. Landsberg, L., and Young, J. B. (1981): Diet-induced changes in sympathoadrenal activity: implications for thermogenesis and obesity. *Obesity and Metab.*, 1:5–33.
31. Lew, E. A. (1961): New data on underweight and overweight persons. *J. Am. Diet. Assoc.*, 38:323–327.
32. Maddox, G. L., Back, K., and Liederman, V. R. (1968): Overweight as a social deviance and disability. *J. Health Soc. Behav.*, 9:287–298.
33. Mann, G. V. (1974): The influence of obesity on health. *N. Engl. J. Med.*, 291:226–232.
34. Marx, J. L. (1981): Natriuretic hormone linked to hypertension. *Science*, 212:1255–1257.
35. Messerli, F. H., Christie, B., DeCarvellio, J. G., et al. (1981): Obesity in essential hypertension. Hemodynamics, intravascular volume, sodium excretion and plasma renin activity. *Arch. Intern. Med.*, 141:81–85.
36. National Center for Health Statistics. (1977): *Weight by height and age of adults 18–74 years: United States, 1971–1974*. Vital and Health Statistics Advance Data No. 14. United States Government Printing Office, Maryland.
37. *National Commission on Diabetes Report, Vol. 3, Part 1*, (1975): D.H.E.W. Publication No. (N.I.H.) 76–1021.
38. Pooling Project Research Group (1978): Relationship of blood pressure, serum cholesterol, smoking habit, relative weight and ECG abnormalities to incidence of major coronary events. Final Report of the Pooling Project. *J. Chronic Dis.*, 31–201.
39. Rabkin, S. W., Mathewson, F. A. L., and Hsu, P. H. (1977): Relation of body weight to development of ischemic heart disease of young North American men after a 26 year observation period: The Manitoba Study. *Am. J. Cardiol.*, 39:452–458.
40. Rimm, A. A., Werner, L. H., Van Yserloo, B., and Bernstein, R. A. (1975): Relationship of obesity and disease in 73,532 weight-conscious women. *Public Health Rep.*, 90:44–51.
41. Rimm, A. A., and White, P. L. (1979): Obesity: Its risks and hazards. In: *Obesity in America*, edited by G. A. Bray, pp. 103–124. N.I.H. Publication No. 79. p. 359.
42. Shurtleff, D. (1974): Some characteristics related to the incidence of cardiovascular disease and death: The Framingham Study, 18-year follow-up. In: *The Framingham Study*, Section 30, edited by W. B. Kannel and T. Gordon. D.H.E.W. Publication No. (N.I.H.) 74, p. 599.
43. Silverstone, J. T., Gordon, R. P., and Stunkard, A. J. (1969): Social factors in obesity in London. *Practitioner*, 202:686–688.
44. Society of Actuaries (1960): *Build and Blood Pressure Study, 1959*. Chicago.
45. Sorlie, P., Gordon, T., and Kannel, W. B. (1980): Body Build and Mortality. *JAMA*, 243:1828–1831.
46. Stamler, J., Rhomberg, P., Schoenberger, J. A., Shekelle, R. B., et al. (1975): Multivariate analysis of the relationship of 7 variates to blood pressure. *J. Chron. Dis.*, 28:527–548.
47. Stamler, J., Stamler, R., Romberg, A., Dyer, A., Berkson, D. M., et al. (1975): Multivariate analysis of the relationship of six variables to blood pressure: Findings from Chicago community surveys 1965–1971. *J. Chron. Dis.*, 28:499–525.

48. Stamler, R., Stamler, J., Reidlinger, W. F., et al. (1978): Weight and blood pressure: Findings in hypertension screening of 1 million Americans. *JAMA*, 240:1607–1620.
49. Strauss, J. R., and Wise, L. (1978): Operative risks of obesity. *Surgery*, 146:286–291.
50. Stunkard, A. J. (1975): Obesity and the social environment. In: *Recent Advances in Obesity Research*, pp. 178–190. Newman Publishing, London.
51. Stunkard, A. J., D'Aquili, E., Fox, S., and Filion, R. D. L. (1972): The influence of social class on obesity and thinness in children. *JAMA*, 22:579–584.
52. Tobian, L. (1978): Hypertension and obesity. *N. Engl. J. Med.*, 298:46.
53. Whitelaw, G. L. (1971): Association of social class and sibling number with skinfold thickness in London schoolboys. *Hum. Biol.*, 43:414–420.

Health and Obesity, edited by H. L. Conn, Jr.,
E. A. DeFelice, and P. Kuo. Raven Press,
New York © 1983.

Biochemistry and Development of Adipose Tissue in Man

Rudolph L. Leibel, *Elliot M. Berry, and Jules Hirsch

*Laboratory of Human Behavior and Metabolism, Rockefeller University,
New York, New York 10021*

ROLE OF ADIPOSE TISSUE IN ENERGY BALANCE

The triglyceride molecule is a solution to the biological requirement for a high density (potential chemical energy per unit weight), low entropy form of chemical energy storage. The highly reduced carbon atoms of its component fatty acids, provide a potential energy concentration of approximately 7 kcal/g in human adipose tissue. The hydrophobic nature of triglyceride enables energy storage with insignificant osmotic load and in relatively low density (weight per volume). This compares with an effective energy concentration of 0.8 kcal/g of wet muscle protein and 1.0 kcal/g of wet hepatic or muscle glycogen. Table 1 details the distribution of stored calories in the tissues of a healthy 70-kg male. The substitution of glycogen for the 105,000 kcal usually stored as triglyceride would more than double the body weight of an adult male. The ability to use the components of triglyceride (glycerol and free fatty acids) in various metabolic processes allows higher organisms to survive prolonged food deprivation without extensive protein catabolism, or central nervous system impairment due to glucose deprivation. Free fatty acids are used as fuel by myocardium, skeletal muscle, and liver and can be converted in the liver

TABLE 1. *Energy-storage sites in a 70-kg man*

Fuel	Tissue	Grams	kcal
Triglyceride	Adipose	15,000	105,000
Glycogen	Liver	70	280
	Muscle	120	480
Glucose	Body fluids	20	80
Protein	Muscle	6,000	25,000

*On sabbatical leave from the Department of Medicine B, Hadassah University Hospital, Jerusalem, Israel 91120

(under appropriate endocrinologic and nutritional circumstances) to water soluble ketones, which may serve as fuel for the brain as well as muscle and liver. The glycerol is used as a substrate for hepatic gluconeogenesis (119) and is a major source of glucose during starvation.

Adipose tissue is a collection of adipocytes or fat storage cells with highly specialized biochemical capabilities as briefly described below. Among invertebrates, only arthropods display a distinct adipose organ, and among vertebrates, well-developed subcutaneous adipose tissue appears only in homeotherms (152). In addition to so-called "white" adipose tissue (WAT), some mammals also have "brown" adipose tissue (BAT), which derives its color from the cytochrome pigment of its densely packed mitochondria. BAT is located in distinct anatomic sites (mainly in the mediastinum and around the kidneys) in various rodents, hibernators, and the human neonate (45,105). It is now believed (see below) that a specialized mitochondrial membrane component of BAT is able to release substrate energy directly as heat rather than storing it in the high-energy phosphate bonds of ATP. This capability is used to "warm up" torpid hibernating animals, to produce nonshivering thermogenesis in human neonates and some rodents, and to allow facultative "burning off" of excess caloric intake in rats, possibly by producing diet-induced thermogenesis (64,130). The role of BAT in thermogenesis in adult man is uncertain, but is currently under investigation.

LONG-TERM CONTROL OF BODY WEIGHT

Long-term shifts in the body weight of adults are mainly dependent on changes in adipose tissue stores. The net systemic balance between caloric intake and caloric expenditure (as basal metabolic processes, physical activity, and possibly nonshivering thermogenesis) ultimately determines the quantity of fat stored by the organism. There is a large amount of literature that indicates that energy stores in animals are regulated over long periods of time and that this control is achieved by interacting processes involving both food intake and energy expenditure (26). In man, long-term energy balance is clearly under the influence of a complex of psychological and environmental factors (24). However, the relative constancy of body weight over time (42, 70, 151), despite wide fluctuations in caloric intake (111, 137), suggests that internal homeostatic systems play a role in this process as well. Control of body weight is not entirely analogous to those processes regulating circulating glucose and calcium levels, or plasma pH, in that the upper level limit appears to vary widely between individuals and the resistance to downward deflections of adipose mass is, in general, greater than the counterregulatory forces opposing deposition of excess adipose tissue. Such a control mechanism would have considerable survival value because extra calories could be stored as fat during periods of plentiful food supply, whereas energy conserving processes would be invoked early during food deprivation (104).

A critical issue concerning long-term energy homeostasis is precisely which variables are being regulated. Adipose tissue could, by analogy to an electric circuit, be either "in parallel" or "in series" with processes tending to hold systemic energy balance approximately constant. In the former circumstance, adipose tissue mass would simply reflect passively the organismic net long-term energy balance but would play no direct role in influencing this balance. If, however, adipose tissue were in series with the regulatory process, it might influence net energy balance by any one of a number of mechanisms, e.g., (a) varying rates of intrinsic energy-consuming processes related to glyceride synthesis and breakdown, (b) releasing free fatty acids and glycerol so as to affect plasma concentrations, which in turn would influence brain "feeding centers," and (c) influencing plasma levels of insulin, other peptide hormones, or catecholamine turnover rates, which might, in turn, affect food intake and energy expenditure. At present it is uncertain whether any of the above possibilities are significant elements in energy homeostasis in man. In order to evaluate any possibility, some understanding of the biochemistry of the adipocyte is essential. The following section is a brief review of biochemical aspects of adipocyte function relevant to a consideration of adipose tissue as an "in series" regulator of energy storage.

BASIC BIOCHEMISTRY OF ADIPOSE TISSUE

White Adipose Tissue

Although WAT functions as a thermal insulator and mechanical cushion, its major role is as a buffer for imbalances in energy intake relative to systemic energy requirements. Accordingly, the biochemistry of this tissue is designed to synthesize and store triglycerides during periods of positive energy balance and to release this chemical energy to distant organs via the circulation during periods of relative deficiency of caloric intake. The constant possibility of brief starvation or brief surfeit requires an active metabolism even under eucaloric conditions, when energy needs are precisely met by intake.

Figure 1 illustrates the process by which glycerides are synthesized and released by adipose tissue. Fatty acids are made available to the adipocyte in the form of triglycerides or as free fatty acids (FFA) bound to albumin. These fatty acids are either ingested in the diet or synthesized by the liver. Adipocytes of adult human beings synthesize relatively little FFA (65, 121) when compared with hepatic synthesis or synthesis rates in the adipose tissue of growing rats. Triglycerides represent the quantitatively most significant source of fatty acids for esterification by adipose tissue since this is the form in which dietary lipids are ultimately "packaged" by the gut and liver. Triglycerides in the form of chylomicrons (intestinal absorption) or lipoproteins (hepatic synthesis) are hydrolyzed to component glycerol and FFA by lipoprotein lipase (LPL), which is formed in the adipocyte and secreted into adjacent endothelial cells. Both chylomicrons and very low density lipoproteins (the major transport vehicle to adipose tissue of fatty acids synthesized by the liver) contain C-II apoprotein, which is a specific activator of LPL (99). Triglycerides cross the capillary endothelium and are hydrolyzed in the endothelium and in the

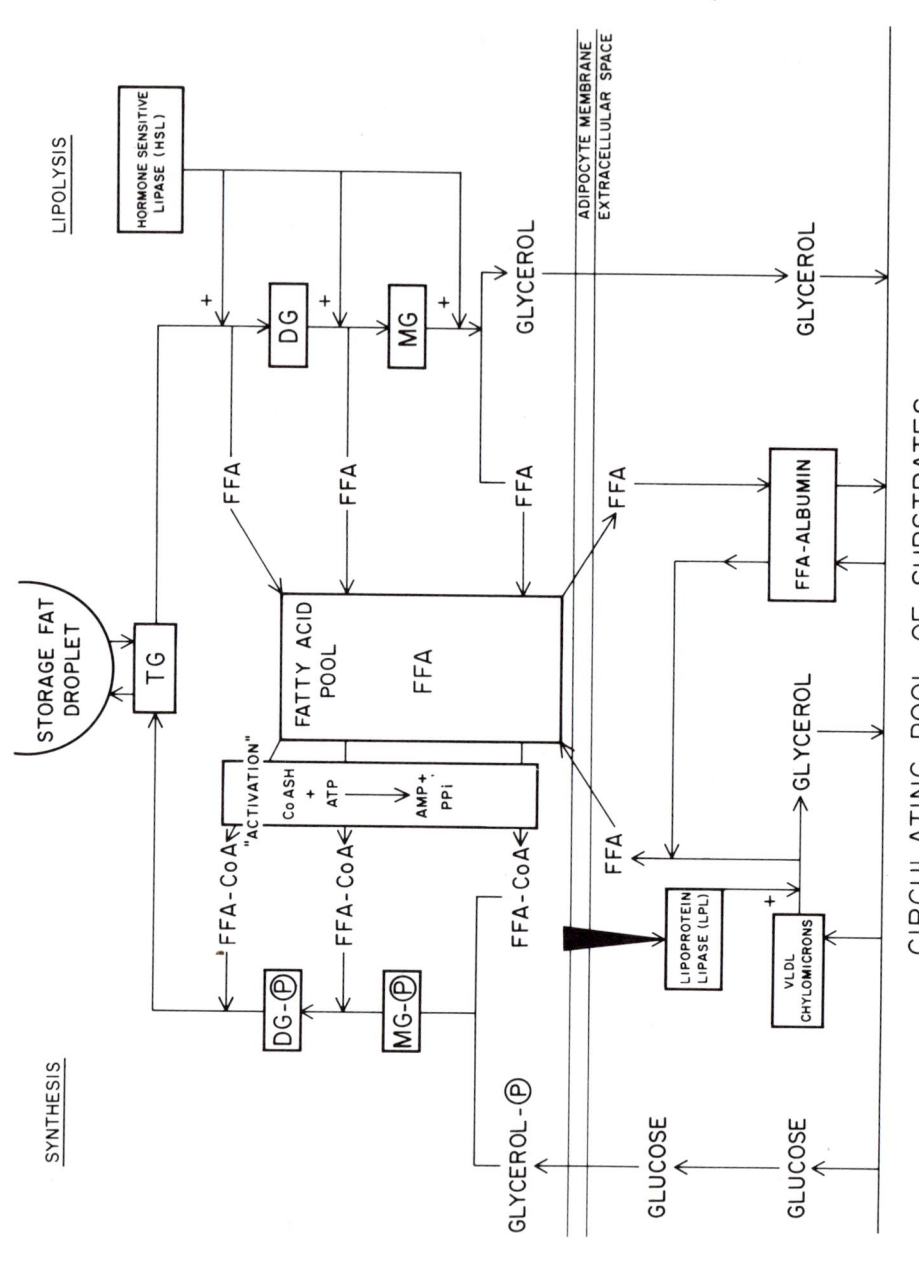

CIRCULATING POOL OF SUBSTRATES

subendothelial space (133, 134). The fatty acids released by this process are taken up by adipocytes in a concentration-dependent fashion by a transmembrane transport protein (1) and rapidly reesterified to triglyceride using glucose-derived glycerol 3-phosphate as ·the source of glyceride-glycerol. Since adipose tissue (unlike liver) has only very low levels of glycerol kinase, the glycerol released by LPL hydrolysis of glycerides cannot be used by adipose tissue and is thus returned to the circulation (154). Glycerides are synthesized mainly in cytoplasmic and mitochondrial sites (4), but there is some recent evidence to suggest that such synthesis may occur in the plasma membrane as well (63). It has been suggested that newly synthesized glycerides are transported as "liposomes" to the large central lipid droplet (4). However this process occurs, newly synthesized di- and triglycerides are preferentially released by lipolytic stimuli in both rat and human adipose tissue for only a brief time. That is, for a matter of minutes or at most hours, the last glycerides synthesized are among the first to be hydrolyzed during lipolysis (115, 161). Thereafter, all lipids behave as though they were stored in a single, very slowly turning over, compartment.

Adipose tissue does not release whole glycerides into the bloodstream. Rather, the central lipid droplet is acted upon by a multienzyme complex (hormone sensitive lipase, HSL), which hydrolyzes the constituent triglycerides to FFA and glycerol (135). Although the resulting glycerol cannot be reutilized by the adipocyte and is therefore released at a rate proportional to the rate of triglyceride hydrolysis, some of the FFA react with endogenous glycerol phosphate to form triglycerides. The fraction of fatty acids that is reesterified in this way, and thus the relative rates of efflux of FFA and glycerol from adipocytes, is dependent on such interrelated factors as the nutritional status of the individual, plasma substrate and hormone levels, and the rate of glycolysis within the adipose tissue (112).

Nonesterified or FFA circulate tightly bound to albumin (67). Under ordinary circumstances FFA comprise only approximately 2% of total plasma lipids. How-

---

FIG. 1. A diagrammatic representation of glyceride metabolism in the adipocyte. Triglyceride (TG) is synthesized from fatty acid molecules esterified onto a glycerol-$\textcircled{P}$ backbone. The glycerol-$\textcircled{P}$ is derived from circulating glucose; the fatty acid molecules come from circulating FFA as well as the breakdown of dietary chylomicrons and VLDL-TG, mediated through the action of LPL synthesized and secreted by the adipocyte. The glycerol molecules released by hydrolysis of TG are returned to the circulation since adipocytes—lacking glycerol kinase—cannot utilize them as substrates for new glyceride synthesis. Inside the cell, FFA molecules appear to enter a common pool consisting of both incoming and outgoing fatty acids. In the synthetic pathway fatty acids must first form a thioester with CoA before reacting with glycerol-$\textcircled{P}$ to yield, in a stepwise fashion, MG-$\textcircled{P}$, DG-$\textcircled{P}$, and finally TG. TG is stored in the central fat droplet and is sequentially degraded by the action of the HSL enzyme complex, which is, in turn, regulated by cyclic AMP. FFA molecules thus released enter the common pool where they may undergo reesterification, metabolic degradation (beta-oxidation), or release into the circulation as substrates for liver, skeletal, and cardiac muscle. Insulin promotes TG storage by stimulating the uptake of glucose and fatty acids, the formation of LPL, and also by reducing lipolysis through inhibition of HSL activity. Abbreviations: MG, DG, TG: Mono-, di-, triglyceride; FFA: free fatty acids; VLDL: very low density lipoproteins; MG-$\textcircled{P}$: lysophosphatidic acid; DG-$\textcircled{P}$: phosphatidic acid; glycerol-$\textcircled{P}$: glycerol phosphate; ATP: adenosine triphosphate; CoA-SH: coenzyme A; PPi: pyrophosphate.

ever, their short plasma half-life (2 to 3 min) and high turnover rates (100 to 400 g/24 hr depending on the duration of fasting) provide a substantial contribution to systemic energy requirements (800 to 3,200 kcal/24 hr) (69, 101). Cardiac muscle uses FFA as fuel almost exclusively; liver and exercising skeletal muscle also rely substantially on FFA as a source of substrate for oxidation (118, 160).

As this description of WAT biochemistry implies, triglyceride synthesis and hydrolysis are not mutually exclusive processes. In fact, it is their simultaneous activity and mutual sensitivity to various hormones and metabolites discussed below that accounts for the organism's ability to regulate FFA release from adipose tissue with a high degree of precision. The integration of these processes and the control of the relative preponderance of one over the other, are achieved by the level of substrate availability and the action of the endocrine system (Table 2). LPL levels in adipose tissue are directly proportional to circulating insulin levels as well as to adipocyte size (125). HSL activity is ultimately regulated by a cyclic AMP-dependent protein kinase (34, 78). The human adipocyte membrane has beta-1 (lipolysis) and alpha-2 (antilipolysis) adrenoceptors that influence HSL activity by reciprocal effects on intracellular cyclic AMP levels (32, 142). There is also an alpha-1 receptor that regulates membrane phosphatidyl inositol turnover and movement of extracellular calcium into the cytosol (53); shifts in intracellular calcium may, in turn, act as a "second messenger" for regulatory enzymes similar to the function of cyclic AMP (37). Epinephrine (mainly of adrenal origin) and norepinephrine (mainly from autonomic nerve endings) are the two major naturally occurring agonists for this adrenoceptor system. Although their relative potencies at specific alpha and beta receptors are somewhat different, each has the ability to stimulate both types of receptor (107). The net response of adipose tissue (lipolysis or antilipolysis) to stimulation by one of these mixed agonists is in most circumstances a reflection of the relative preponderance of beta versus alpha receptors in the plasma membrane. This balance is, in turn, influenced by adipocyte size (66, 117), site (116, 143), the subject's age and nutritional status (31), and levels of thyroid hormone (129) and cortisol (68, 135).

The relevance of these opposing adrenoceptors to the systemic economy of lipids is an unresolved issue. Prolonged fasting causes a several-fold increase in basal

TABLE 2. *A comparison of the properties of the two major enzyme systems regulating triglyceride synthesis and release in adipose tissue*

	Lipoprotein lipase	Hormone-sensitive lipase
Site of action	Extracellular (capillary endothelium)	Intracellular
Function	Promotes triglyceride storage	Promotes lipolysis
Substrate	Chylomicrons, VLDL	Fat droplet
Insulin	Induces and activates	Inhibits
Epinephrine	Inhibits	Activates (β-adrenoceptor)
Cyclic AMP	Inhibits	Activates

lipolysis rate, which is poorly suppressible *in vivo* (98) or *in vitro (unpublished observations)* by the administration of a beta adrenergic blocking agent such as propranolol. In addition, fasting causes an augmented alpha-2 receptor activity of human adipose tissue *in vitro* as shown by antilipolysis on exposure to epinephrine (5, 31). Yet, the systemic infusion of epinephrine into semi-fasted individuals produces accelerated lipolysis rather than causing antilipolysis *(unpublished observations)*. Finally, the autonomic nerve supply to WAT appears to be limited to the vascular system supplying the tissue. Unlike BAT, there is no apparent direct innervation of parenchymal adipocytes. Thus, some portion of autonomic nervous influence on WAT function may be mediated by effects on blood flow (43). There is still considerable uncertainty as to the degree to which *in vitro* studies of adipose tissue reflect *in vivo* functions.

Although pharmacologic concentrations of various peptides (growth hormone, ACTH, glucagon) will cause *in vitro* lipolysis in rat adipose tissue (135), insulin appears to be a more significant regulator of adipose tissue function. Insulin both increases glucose entry and hence glycerol phosphate availability for triglyceride synthesis and inhibits HSL activity, thereby decreasing FFA release (90). Although insulin can lower cyclic AMP induced by lipolytic hormones (35), its effects on lipolysis can be demonstrated at concentrations that do not affect intracellular levels of cyclic AMP (92). Shapiro has suggested (135) that insulin may influence a subpool of cyclic AMP critical to lipolysis but so small that significant shifts in its activity are not detectable against the background activity of this compound in other compartments of the cell. The nonlinear relationship between intracellular cyclic AMP levels and rates of hormone-stimulated lipolysis may be due to a similar phenomenon (6, 59, 91).

The relative activities of HSL and LPL are probably important determinants of the net balance of calories stored in adipose tissue (Table 2). Insulin influences this relationship by direct reciprocal influences on the activity of these enzymes. There are, in addition, intrinsic control loops within adipose tissue due to the inhibitory effects of intracellular FFA on both LPL and HSL activity: (a) The reesterification of a portion of the FFA resulting from stimulated lipolysis consumes ATP, which could otherwise be used in protein (LPL) synthesis (122). Thus, stimulation of HSL leads indirectly to a reduction of LPL activity. (b) Intracellular accumulation of FFA inhibits *in vitro* lipolysis in adipose tissue (127). This inhibition is accompanied by a lowering of cyclic AMP accumulation, which may be due to consumption of ATP in the reesterification process (33). Inhibition of lipolysis by intracellular FFA protects the cell against the detergent effects of high concentrations of FFA and prevents the release to the circulation of FFA in excess of those required for current metabolic needs.

Brown Adipose Tissue

It is generally agreed that BAT is a major thermogenic tissue. BAT resembles WAT in that it uses the same biochemical pathways to store and release fatty acids.

However, unlike WAT, these fatty acids are involved locally in heat generation rather than for use as substrate at distant sites. In rodents the vascular supply to BAT is greater per unit weight of tissue than that of any other organ (58). This allows rapid substrate delivery as well as heat transfer. The tissue has a very rich sympathetic nerve supply, which innervates both the arterial blood vessels and parenchymal cells (46). The cytoplasmic lipid stores of BAT are multilocular and surrounded by a large number of mitochondria, which are packed with cristae (147). According to the chemiosmotic theory of mitochondrial function (83, 109), the chemical energy released during cytochrome electron transport is stored as potential energy in protons pumped out of the mitochondrial matrix. The energy released by the movement of these protons back into the matrix is used to form ATP. The mitochondria of BAT (Fig. 2) contain proton uniports (32,000 Dalton protein) on the outer face of the inner mitochondrial membrane that are inhibited by the high affinity binding of purine nucleotides (113). FFA released during autonomic (nor-

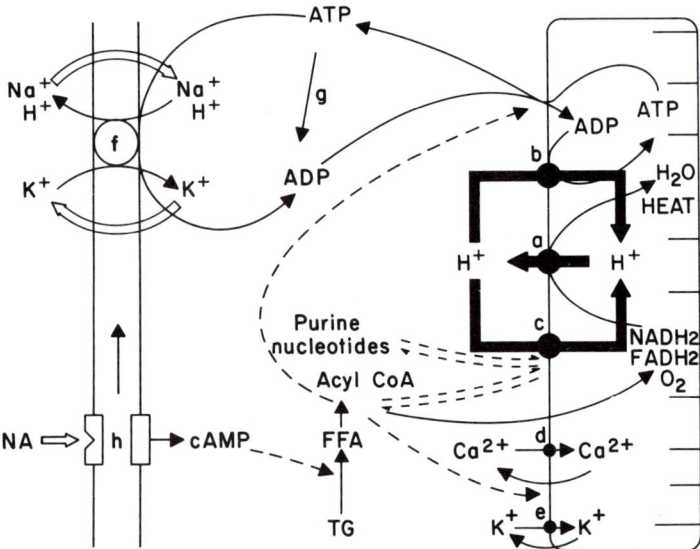

FIG. 2. Mechanisms of thermogenesis, with particular reference to nonshivering thermogenesis in BAT. The intracellular locations of the following processes are **(a)** electron transport system of inner mitochondrial membrane, responsible for oxidation of reduced coenzymes (NADH$_2$, FADH$_2$) and pumping of H$^+$ across the membrane to create the proton electrochemical gradient; **(b)** ATP synthesis (oxidative phosphorylation) driven by the proton electrochemical gradient; **(c)** proton conductance pathway, responsible for allowing the dissipation of the proton electrochemical gradient without the simultaneous synthesis of ATP; **(d)** calcium uptake and release; **(e)** potassium uptake and release; **(f)** Na$^+$, K$^+$ ATPase (Na$^+$ pump) in the plasma membrane; **(g)** other ATPases located in cytosol or other cellular constituents, e.g., myosin ATPase of myofibrils (arrows between ADP and ATP on sides of inner membrane denote the adenine nucleotide translocase); **(h)** site of action of norepinephrine on its receptor in the plasma membrane, which results in adenylate cyclase activation to form cyclic AMP (cAMP) and changes in permeability to Na$^+$ and K$^+$ (denoted by arrow in membrane). Dashed lines illustrate regulatory effects of purine nucleotides (they bind to the proton conductance pathway, site c, to inhibit conductance) and of acyl CoA (they displace purine nucleotides from the proton conductance translocase). (From Himms-Hagen, ref. 81, with permission.)

epinephrine) stimulated lipolysis displace the nucleotides from the ion uniports, allowing protons to "leak back" to the mitochondrial matrix without being coupled to ATP synthesis (79). Mitochondrial membrane purine binding capacity correlates well with BAT thermogenic activity, being increased in newborn guinea pigs, awakening hibernators and cold-adapted rats (77, 81). The potential energy represented by the protons that have been "pumped" out of the matrix is thus lost as heat rather than being stored in a phosphoanhydride bond of ATP. This is, apparently, the major mechanism for heat production in BAT. Contributory thermogenic processes may also include increased pumping of Na^+ and K^+ by Na^+, K^+-ATPase (86). Electrical stimulation of the hypothalamus in the region of the ventromedial nucleus (an area subserving eating behavior and autonomic regulation) increases triglyceride turnover (136) and heat production (123) in BAT but not WAT. Thus, an area of the brain that is important in regulating food intake also appears to influence the efficiency with which the ingested calories are used.

BAT and WAT are histologically similar in the newborn infant (110), but BAT either disappears or is transformed into WAT with increasing age (149). It seems possible but it is not proven that some nonshivering thermogenesis in the neonate and in the older human being is mediated by cells that morphologically resemble white adipocytes but contain mitochondria with the energy-dissipating ion uniports. Diminished *in vitro* heat production of white adipocytes from obese as compared to normal weight individuals (144) could be due to a defect in the mitochondrial system described above. There is need for studies of the 32,000 Dalton uniport regulator in the membranes of human WAT mitochondria obtained from individuals at various ages and degrees of adiposity.

DEVELOPMENT OF ADIPOSE TISSUE

Basic Concepts

Organ growth occurs in three synchronized but overlapping phases—hyperplasia, hyperplasia–hypertrophy, and hypertrophy. The timing of these phases varies between organs and species. Studies by Winick and Noble (158, 159) demonstrated that organ cellularity could be altered by early nutritional experience: under- and overfeeding during periods of cellular hyperplasia resulted in permanent respective decreases and increases in cellularity of organs normally showing hyperplastic growth during this period. Returning to normal food intake after a period of deprivation normalized cell size but did not rectify changes in organ cellularity. These findings led to the concept of "sensitive periods"—ontogenic time windows for each organ during which the plane of nutrition could permanently influence the cellularity of an organ (48). Knittle and Hirsch (96) extended these findings to the adipose organ, showing that the cellularity of rat epididymal fat pads could be permanently altered by preweaning nutrition: rats raised in large (22 pups) litters had fewer epididymal adipocytes than those raised in small (4 pups) litters. Subsequent studies have shown that, in comparison to animals reared in a medium-sized (8 to 10 pups) litter, small litter animals show approximately a 20% increase in cell number as adults whereas large litter animals have approximately a 26% reduction in adipose organ cellularity as adults (88). Thus, in rodents, over- and underfeeding during the suckling period creates reciprocal changes in adipose organ cellularity. Since glucose metabolism (combustion of CO_2, glyceride formation) on a per cell basis remains unchanged, net glyceride synthesis is greater in those animals with more cells. These findings, and the observation that increased adipocyte number (rather than size) was primarily responsible for the increased size of the fat organ in extremely obese adult human beings (84), led to the formulation of the so-called "fat cell hypothesis" of obesity whose fundamental tenets may be stated as follows: (a) early overstimulation leads to permanent hyperplasia of the adipose organ; (b) this hyperplastic organ, by virtue of normal per cell metabolic performance and a tendency to maintain a "normal" volume of lipid in each adipocyte, obligates a greater fraction of substrate intake to disposition in the fat organ thus causing and perpetuating obesity. Corollaries bearing on the ontogeny and possible prevention of human obesity were immediately drawn, and studies begun to define more precisely the development of the adipose organ in both animals and man.

This hypothesis was a natural result of the growing understanding of the very active metabolism within adipocytes and of the suggestion that adipose organ mass might be a regulated variable in the complex of systems that achieve energy balance. The adipocyte thus moved from its prior conceptual position as a passive monitor of long-term nutritional status into a critical role in the regulation of the mass of the adipose organ. Although the validity of this concept has never been conclusively demonstrated, it has had a substantial impact on strategies in obesity research. In clinical medicine this has been manifest in efforts both to demonstrate correlations between obesity in early life and adulthood and to prevent this theoretically presumed concordance by early nutritional interventions. Animal studies have focused on demonstrating regulation of adipose organ mass by both feedback systems between adipocytes and appetitive behavior, and mutable intrinsic characteristics of adipocytes, e.g., LPL levels or insulin receptors. Pharmacologic studies in both animal models and man have examined the possible role of adrenergic receptor systems in regulating adipocyte size. Tissue culture methods have been applied to the study of adipose tissue in an effort to elucidate the temporal characteristics and biochemical processes of adipocyte formation and differentiation.

Methods of Study

Below, we discuss the methods which are currently most widely employed in the study of human adipose tissue. Further details may be obtained in a recent review (73).

Cell Counting Within Specific Adipose Depots or Subcutaneous Sites

Cell counting involves either direct measurement (by eye piece micrometer or particle size analyzer) of cell diameter in frozen cut or paraffin-embedded sections of adipose tissue, or the counting of isolated osmium-fixed or unfixed cells by Coulter Counter or by direct observation. With the microscopic technique, cell volume is frequently converted to weight by assuming the cell to have the density of triolein (0.915 g/ml). With some cell counting methods, a piece of tissue from the same site is chemically extracted to determine lipid content per unit wet weight of tissue. Measurement of cell number and lipid content per unit wet weight allows the calculation of lipid content per cell. Automated methods for the direct measurement of the size of adipocytes are currently available (41, 140, 146).

Debate continues in regard to the relative merits of these various methods (8, 21, 89, 155). The osmium-fixation method of Hirsch and Gallian (85), probably the most widely employed, has the virtues of objectivity, large numbers of cells counted, and the potential (by adjusting the electronic "gate") to generate a cell-size frequency distribution. Potential problems with the method include the cost and toxicity of osmium tetroxide and the fact that cells with diameters less than 25 microns are excluded by the filtration process that precedes the actual cell counting. Opponents of the osmium fixation method (8, 94, 155) have maintained that this inability to detect very small (or immature) adipocytes leads to underestimates of cellularity in depots containing small cells (or pockets of small cells) and to misdesignation as tissue hyperplasia of the phenomenon of lipid filling of preexisting adipocytes to a volume sufficient to raise them above the detection threshold of the method. This issue appears to be of minimal relevance in the assessment of adipocyte cellularity in adult man where even extensive weight reduction and associated marked decreases in mean adipocyte size do not result in any decrease in apparent cellularity (84). The close correlations between ontogeny of the adipose organ as reflected in the osmium fixation cell counting method and DNA labeling techniques (see below) further suggests that the error introduced by the omission of cells less than 25 microns in diameter is small. This may be due to rapid lipid filling of newly formed adipocytes, leaving few very small unfilled "preadipocytes" in the tissue at any given time (14).

Intact tissue methods are labor intensive, tedious, and subject to errors in the conversion of measures of polyhedral cells to spherical volumes. Nonetheless, these methods have the advantage of allowing direct visualization of the disposition of single cells or groups of cells within a section of the tissue. This may be important in assessing the cellularity of very immature fat depots. In the final analysis, as both Brooke (28) and Bjorntorp (22) have emphasized, there is a remarkable uniformity of results achieved by workers using a wide range of methodologies.

Regardless of the specific cell sizing method employed, extrapolations to total body fat cell count require the consideration of several other factors: (a) a single sample from a given site may be taken as representative of the site as a whole, with an intrasite variation of approximately 10%, which is no larger than the error of the method (140). (b) The site-to-site variations of adipocyte size *within an individual* are large. Bjorntorp reports that the mean difference between largest and smallest fat cell volume for all examined sites (epigastric, hypogastric, femoral, gluteal, and hip) in 50 consecutive obese women, was 35.6 ± 7.6% of the mean fat cell size for all sites examined (14). Assuming a symmetrical distribution of this fluctuation about the mean value, the error in cell size estimation for an individual introduced by the use of one site as opposed to a multiple site average is approximately 18%. This calculation clearly indicates the desirability of sampling several sites when determining fat cell size in an individual. That site-to-site variation in cell size is the largest single source of variance in estimates of total body fat cell number is indicated in Sjostrom's report of repeat estimates of adipocyte cellularity in 11 obese and nonobese weight-stable patients (138). The 12.2% coefficient of variation obtained when only hypogastric region cell weight is measured is reduced to 6.2% when a 4-site mean is used. This error for group means is smaller than the 18% error for interindividual comparisons, which is due mainly to regional variation in fat cell size. There may also be ethnic differences in regional adipose cell sizes: Scandinavian investigators (13, 141) report no significant size differences between gluteal and hypogastric adipocytes whereas some American workers (40, 132) find that gluteal adipose cells are significantly larger than those in the hypogastric region. Finally, gluteal adipocytes appear to have the highest correlation ($r = 0.76$) with total body fat and are, therefore, recommended for use in calculating total adipocyte number if only a single site must be used (40). (c) Sex has a clear influence on adipocyte size in rodents, with females having larger fat cells than males (73). In human subjects, although there are fewer data, females appear to have a larger *average* cell size in subcutaneous depots, although within depots men have smaller femoral cells and women smaller epigastric cells (73). Larger gluteal cells in the female may be due in part to hormonal factors as indicated by the finding of specific enlargement of these cells in men treated with estrogens for carcinoma of the prostate (14). There is an age-related trend toward increasing adipocyte size in all depots in both men and women (14). (d) The subcutaneous adipose tissue in man comprises 80 to 90% of the total body fat (10). Most of the remaining fat is located intraabdominally. These visceral fat cells are, in general, smaller than those of the subcutaneous depots and there is a strong correlation between intra- and extraabdominal fat masses in normal weight individuals (23). Some have suggested that failure to enumerate these intraabdominal cells because of their inaccessibility in clinical circumstances could result in an underestimation of total body fat cellularity, particularly in normal weight individuals (89). Bjorntorp and Sjostrom cogently argue against this possibility and suggest that failure to sample visceral adipose tissue directly does not introduce a limiting error into the assessment of total body adipocyte number (21). (e) In order to calculate total body adipocyte number from average lipid weight per cell, one must obtain a measure of total body fat weight either by determining the body density (underwater weighing), multiple-site skinfold thickness (50), or subtraction of lean body mass (estimated from total body water by 40K counting or isotope dilution) from total body weight. Although underwater weighing is probably the most accurate method, it is neither widely available nor applicable in children. Skinfold thickness measures give reliable estimates except in grossly obese individuals in whom accurate measures cannot be obtained due to mechanical problems in the use of calipers. The isotope dilution method gives measures of body water with a precision of 2%, but the conversion of the value to lean body mass, based on an assumed 72.5% water content in lean body mass, is subject to further error, if the water content of lean body mass is not the same for all subjects (120). In fact, this is a major issue in the measurement of lean body mass in infancy and early childhood. In adult man the so-called Pace-Rathbun formula appears to give good agreement with other independent measures of lean body mass.

Cell Culture

Both mature adipocytes and proliferating/differentiating cells from adipose tissue can be sustained or grown in tissue culture. Use of a standardized preparation, such as the 3T3-L1 line of fibroblasts from mouse embryos that develop into adipocytes in tissue culture, permits assessment of local biochemical and plasma factors that may influence adipocyte synthesis and maturation (71). The stromovascular fraction of both rodent and human adipose tissue can be shown to contain cells that will develop in culture into cells having all the biochemical characteristics of adipocytes (15). The number of cells developing into adipocytes appears to be inversely related to the developmental age of the organism studied (3, 14). By making the culture medium viscous with methyl cellulose, the proliferation of new cells is prevented while existing preadipocytes[1] are allowed to continue filling with lipid (18). Use of this technique in parallel with standard culture methods allows the quantification of the relative contributions of new cell synthesis, as compared with preadipocyte filling, to the appearance of mature adipocytes. It has been shown, using such procedures, that rat adipose tissue stromovascular fraction, regardless of the age of the donor, will proliferate to form a cell monolayer in culture. However, the proportion of cells differentiating into mature adipocytes generally declines with increasing age of the donor (18, 19). These findings are somewhat at variance with *in vivo* DNA results (72), which indicate a cessation of adipocyte precursor pro-liferation in rats at 3 to 5 weeks of age. Although Sjostrom has suggested several possible explanations for this discrepancy (138), its existence counsels caution in the over-interpretation of data obtained by either method. Current tissue culture techniques are surely susceptible to confounding artifacts that may diminish the validity of extrapolation to *in vivo* processes, yet much is now being learned about the histogenesis and differentiation of adipose tissue by the use of this technique.

Development of Adipose Tissue in Man

Brown Adipose Tissue

In man, during the first decade of life, BAT with morphologic evidence of biochemical activity (coarsely granular cytoplasm, partial depletion of multilocular

---

[1]The preadipocyte is a cell, having the enzymatic capabilities of an adipocyte, which is destined to become a unilocular adipocyte. Such cells range in diameter from 15 to 30 microns.

fat stores) is found in a wide anatomic distribution. Over the ensuing years this tissue gradually takes on morphologic characteristics of WAT and disappears, first from more peripheral sites (interscapular and anterior abdominal wall) and more gradually from deeper locations (para-aortic, perirenal, suprarenal) (80, 150). The ontogeny of this tissue, as well as its apparent morphologic activation in clinical circumstances of thermal stress (150), is consistent with a role in human thermogenesis at least during certain periods of life. Whereas a congenital derangement in the biochemistry of this tissue has been implicated in a specific rodent (ob/ob mouse) obesity (82), and there have been substantial efforts to extrapolate these findings to energy balance in humans (87), the evidence relating BAT to human obesity must currently be regarded as circumstantial at best.

White Adipose Tissue

In the human fetus, WAT appears between 26 and 30 weeks of gestation. As these cells develop, sudanophilic droplets appear and cell division ceases. These droplets increase in size, ultimately fusing to form a large central core of lipid, forcing the nucleus to the periphery of the cell (95). The neonate has little perirenal or omental fat, but has a subcutaneous fat depot, which represents 10 to 15% of body weight (95). The very high percentage of saturated fatty acids in neonatal triglycerides suggests that most of these fatty acids are synthesized by the fetus from endogenous glucose rather than being obtained by transplacental passage of maternal FFA (10). The average human neonate has 500 g of fat at birth, in cells that each contain approximately 0.120 μg of lipid. Thus, *detectable* adipocyte number is 4.0×10^9. The nonobese adult has about 30×10^9 adipocytes with 0.500 μg of lipid per cell and obese individuals have up to 10^{11} adipocytes with 0.600 to 1.200 μg of lipid per cell (93). Given the fact that early growth of the adipose organ in children involves mainly increases in cell size (44, 97) and that filling of preadipocytes would be expected to increase adipocyte number more than size, the 4- to 25-fold increase in cell number that occurs between birth and adulthood must be due, to some extent, to the production of new adipocytes postpartum.

TABLE 3. *Development of human adipose tissue[a]*

Developmental state	Body weight (kg)	Body weight as fat (%)	Body fat (kg)	Mean fat cell size (μg lipid/cell)	Mean fat cell number ($\times 10^9$)
Neonate	3.2	15	0.48	0.12	4
Child					
1 year	12.5	20	2.50	0.5	5
4 year	20.0	15	3.0	0.5	6
Pre-adolescent	30.0	20	6.0	0.4	15
Adult (nonobese)					
Female	50.0	25–30	15–19	0.4–0.5	30–40
Male	70.0	15–20	14–20	0.4–0.5	28–50
Adult (obese)	100 +	40	40 +	0.6–1.2	60–100

[a]Data from references 38, 39, 52, 75, and 97.

Table 3 summarizes the development of human adipose tissue, and the relationship between cell size and cell number is illustrated in Fig. 3.

Females show a large increase in adiposity at the time of puberty, ultimately reaching a point where fat accounts for approximately 25% of body weight. In addition to the previously noted effect of estrogens on cell size, estrogens may also increase adipocyte number by enhancing the replication of adipocyte precursors (128). Frisch (60, 61) has recently emphasized the interrelationships of body composition and gonadal-axis function in both pubertal and postpubertal females. The mechanisms for this interaction, which may involve aromatization by adipose tissue of circulating androgenic precursors to estrogens (2, 114) or some other "signal" to the hypothalamus from adipose tissue, remain to be elucidated. In males, there is a prepubertal spurt in adiposity, followed by an actual decrease in total body fat during the period of maximal velocity of statural growth during puberty (106). Normal adult males have 15 to 20% of body weight as fat. The greater adiposity of *young* women in comparison to men is the result of a greater number of slightly larger adipocytes. Such differences were not found in a randomly selected group of *middle-aged* men and women (16, 20). During adulthood, adiposity in both males and females increases gradually through a combined process of loss of lean

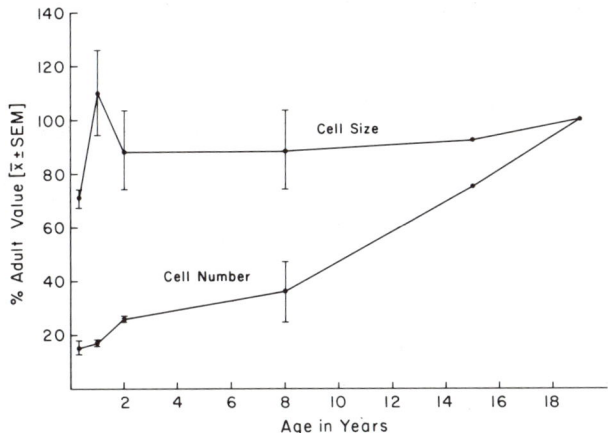

FIG. 3. The relationship between cell size and number of human adipose tissue and chronologic age. Data are taken from short-term longitudinal studies of normal weight individuals by Hager et al. (75) and Knittle et al. (97). The points are plotted as a percentage of adult values (only single values were available at 15 years). It is apparent that, whereas cell size approaches and may even exceed adult levels within the first 2 years of life, cell number increases only slightly during this period. The major increase in cell number occurs around puberty (8 to 15 years). If the data of Knittle et al. (97) on obese individuals (greater than 120% weight/height) are plotted in a similar manner, the pattern of cell size and number development is virtually identical. Therefore, the development of the fat organ in obese patients differs quantitatively but not qualitatively from that of normal individuals. At any given age an obese subject will generally have absolute increases in both cell size and number relative to normal weight controls, but the time course (relative to final obese adult levels of cell size and number) of organ formation is not different from that found in normal weight patients.

body mass and increments in adipose tissue (57). Body weight, however, remains remarkably stable.

THE RELATIVE ROLES OF GENOTYPE AND ENVIRONMENT IN ADIPOSE ORGAN DEVELOPMENT

There is little doubt that both "nature and nurture" contribute variously to specific cases of human obesity. There are discrete syndromes (e.g., Prader-Willi, Alstrom) (27, 102) in which genotype is the apparent predominant factor, and other instances (e.g., adult onset obesity due to overeating and sedentary lifestyle) in which non-genetic factors are clearly predominant. However, the much thornier problem of the relative contributions of genotype and environment to average body composition in man remains unsolved. Twin studies—in which covariance between dizygous twin pairs is used to "factor out" environmental contributions to monozygous twin pair concordance—have indicated a heritability of weight/height or skinfold thickness as high as 0.80 (maximum = 1.0) (25,56). The extent of this heritability increases with age, indicating a progressively more salient expression of genotype against environmental background (29, 156). Further evidence in favor of a substantial contribution of genotype to body composition is provided by a study showing virtually no correlation of weight/height ratios between adopted children and their foster parents or step siblings, despite significant parent to natural offspring and natural sibling correlations for this ratio (12).

On the other hand, certain epidemiologic studies have been interpreted to indicate preponderant environmental influences on body composition (62). And, although some have found a modest correlation between absolute weight or weight gain velocity during the first year of life and the frequency of obesity in childhood (7, 51, 108), others have found that excessive adiposity (by skinfold thickness) in infancy is a very poor predictor of obesity at age 5 years (124). In any event, this relationship weakens with increasing age to the point where some reports show little or no correlation between adiposity in infancy and that occurring in adulthood (148). Additionally, although infant feeding practices (breast versus bottle, timing of introduction of solid foods) may transiently affect adiposity, there is little evidence to support the contention that these practices influence the risk of obesity in the older child or adult (47, 49).

Retrospective studies, such as that of Charney et al. (36), indicate that the obese adult is likely to have been obese in early life. These workers found that infants attaining the 90th percentile for weight in the first 6 months of life had a 2.6-fold increased risk of obesity (greater than 120% ideal weight for height) in adulthood. It is important to note that most obese infants *did not* become obese adults, and that the correlation between infant and adult obesity in no way proves causality. Instances of infant obesity correlated with obesity in adulthood may represent early somatic display of a persistent metabolic diathesis, whereas the more numerous cases of resolving infant obesity may be transient manifestations of environmental forces (e.g., maternal feeding practices).

Another perspective (with possible therapeutic implications) to this problem is provided by studies examining the impact of caloric restriction in infancy on the risk of subsequent obesity. Ravelli et al. (126), reporting on weight/height ratios of 19-year-old males conceived and/or born during the Dutch famine of 1944 to 1945, found a significant decrease in the prevalance of obesity among males exposed to famine during both the last trimester of gestation and first few months of infancy. Undernutrition had to occur during *both* late intrauterine development and early infancy for permanent effects on adipose organ size to occur. The requirement for deprivation during both pregnancy and early life not only implicates a possible "critical period" in human adipose organ development but also may explain why caloric restriction in early infancy alone does not protect against obesity in childhood (138). Finally, caloric restriction and an exercise regimen in 8-year-old obese females failed to diminish an apparently inexorable increase in adipocyte number in some of these patients despite weight loss (76). Such results indicate that although it may be possible in some cases to influence adipocyte formation during some periods of development of obesity, there are other instances in which genetic forces favoring adipocyte production are largely unresponsive to environmental pressures.

Some of the studies described above suggest that, as childhood progresses, multifactorial genetic influences may be more important than environmental factors in determining adiposity. It is important to note that none of the studies implicating genotype in the etiology of obesity indicates the phenotypic pathway(s)—e.g., food intake, adipocyte formation, metabolic efficiency—through which the alleles involved are expressed. Although studies of obese patients have implicated one or another of these processes as preeminent in the etiology of specific cases of severe obesity, the relative contributions of these factors to the adiposity of the general population is unknown. At this point it seems most reasonable to regard human adiposity as a reflection of the interaction of variably predisposing genotypes with a facilitating environment resulting from the ready availability of appetizing foods and reduced need for physical activity. The rising incidence of obesity in the Western world during the past century is due, to some extent, to those improvements in nutrition and hygiene that are also reflected in trends in menarche and greater adult stature. This trend in body composition may be due to environmental enhancement of the population's genetic tendencies to adiposity or the imposition of overfeeding on individuals not otherwise predisposed to obesity, or both. In the latter case it is possible that early childhood feeding practices might predispose some individuals to adult obesity by virtue of permanent anatomic changes in the adipose organ and/or the "programming" of food-related neurochemical responses and behaviors. What is urgently needed is a biochemical or behavioral "marker" that can identify, with high specificity, individuals at risk for obesity. The prospective application of such a test to cohorts of infants subsequently monitored for body composition into adulthood could help solve the critical issue of the relative contributions of nature and nurture to the etiology of obesity in man.

TYPES OF OBESITY DISTINGUISHED BY ADIPOCYTE GEOMETRY

Despite the debates concerning appropriate methodology for determining adipocyte number, the hypercellularity of some obese cannot be dismissed as a technical artifact. In large studies both the Rockefeller (84) and the Swedish groups (20, 139) have demonstrated a positive correlation of fat cell number with total body fat over a range including normal (30 × 10⁹ adipocytes) and extremely obese (100 × 10⁹ adipocytes) individuals. Fat cell size, on the other hand, rises with increasing adiposity to an upper limit of approximately 1.2 microgram lipid/cell, which occurs at approximately 170% ideal weight (84) or 30 kg body fat (138). Beyond these relatively modest levels of obesity, there is little or no further increase in adipocyte size with increasing obesity. Thus, mildly obese individuals may be hypertrophic without being hyperplastic, but the severely obese display both hypertrophy and hyperplasia of fat cells. Normotrophic, hyperplastic obesity is not a naturally occurring phenomena, but may result from weight reduction of a hypertrophic, hyperplastic obese individual. These relationships are summarized in Figs 4, 5, and 6.

It is possible that positive energy balance in adults can result in an increase in adipose organ cellularity, probably by the production of new cells rather than by the filling of preadipocytes (15, 153). However, subsequent dieting and associated decrease in adipocyte size is not likely to be accompanied by a reduction in adipocyte number. Once formed, these cells appear to remain permanently within the adipose organ. Thus, with each episode of weight gain sufficient to cause further adipocyte hyperplasia, the individual permanently increases adipocyte number. Sjostrom has, in fact, reported gradually increasing adipose organ cellularity in obese adult females studied repeatedly over a period of years (138).

There are conflicting reports with regard to the impact of the age of onset of obesity on adipose organ cellularity in later life. Brook et al. (30) reported increased

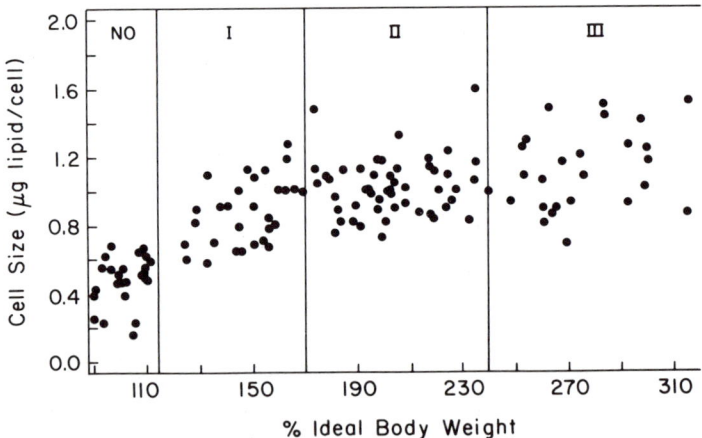

FIG. 4. The relationship between mean adipocyte size (microgram lipid/cell) and degree of obesity [expressed as percent ideal body weight using the Metropolitan Life Insurance Co. Standards (145)]. I, II, and III refer to three groups of subjects with increasing severity of obesity (% ideal body weight). NO: nonobese; I: 110 to 170%; II: 171–240%; III: greater than 240%. Figs. 4, 5, and 6 are based on a study of 106 obese and 25 nonobese patients 30 to 35 years of age. Cell size was calculated as a mean of 3 subcutaneous sites. Body water was determined by tritiated water dilution. (Figs. 4, 5, and 6 from Hirsch and Batchelor, ref. 84, with permission.)

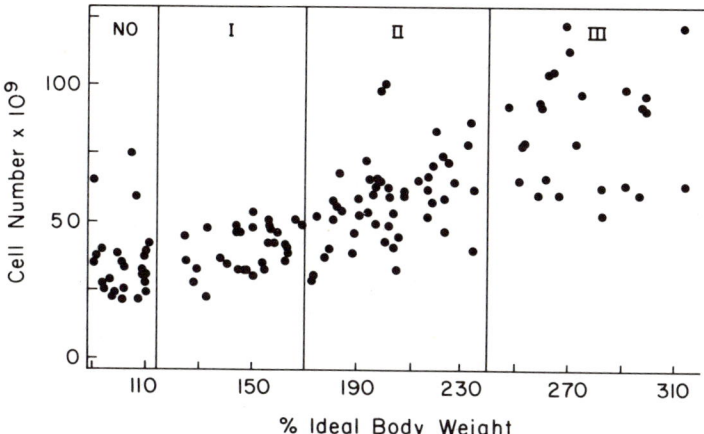

FIG. 5. The relationship between total fat cell number and percent ideal body weight. Cell number was estimated by dividing total body fat by mean cell size. Body fat, in turn, was calculated from the difference between body weight and the lean body mass as determined from the distribution of tritiated water. Groups NO, I, II, and III are described in the legend to Fig. 4.

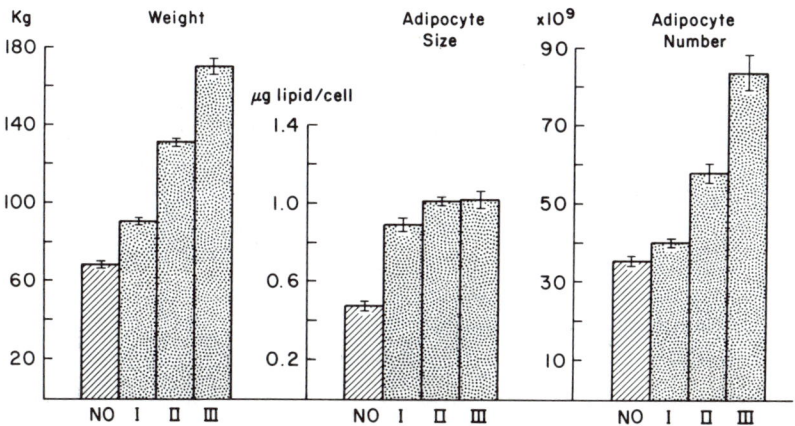

FIG. 6. The relationship (mean ± SEM) of body weight, adipocyte cell size, and adipocyte number in nonobese (NO) individuals and three groups of subjects with increasing severity of obesity. Groups I, II, and III are described in the legend to Fig. 4. Adipocyte cell size and number were calculated as detailed in the legends to Figs. 4 and 5. Of particular interest is the fact that moderate degrees of obesity (to 170% ideal body weight) involve mainly an increase in adipocyte size. Once this maximum size is reached, adipose organ expansion occurs primarily by increases in cell number.

adipose organ cellularity in children who had been obese during the first year of life. However, others (74, 157) have found adipocyte number in obese children of various ages to be unrelated to the age of onset of obesity. In studies of obese adults some groups have reported an apparent relationship between the age of onset of the obesity and the geometry of the fat organ. Individuals with onset of obesity in infancy or childhood are said to be more likely to have hypercellular adipose organs in comparison to nonobese individuals or patients with onset of obesity in adulthood (20, 131). Other workers (9) have found that adipose organ cellularity correlates well with total body fat but not with the age of onset of obesity. Hirsch and Batchelor (84) reported a high correlation between adipocyte number and degree of overweight, but no significant correlation between adipocyte number and age of onset when current adiposity was factored out.

Since the mass of the adipose organ is the product of cell size times cell number, any increase in adipocyte number must be offset by a comparable decrease in adipocyte size if total body fat is to remain constant. Adipocyte size is believed by some investigators to be the variable "regulated" by homeostatic systems subserving long-term organismic energy balance (54, 103). If this hypothesis is correct, then the size of newly formed adipocytes will be regulated to some organismic mean regardless of adipocyte number. Physiologically "blind" to adipocyte number, the organism may seek to hold mean adipocyte volume (rather than total adipose mass or number) at some normative value. An obvious corollary of this hypothesis is that increasing hyperplasticity will lead to increasing intractability to therapy since even at normal adipocyte cell size the hyperplastic obese will have an excess of adipose tissue.

There are, in fact, differences in the response of hyperplastic and hypertrophic forms of obesity to diet treatment. There is a positive correlation between adipocyte number and the absolute amount of weight lost and a negative correlation between adipocyte number and the length of time the reduced weight is maintained (100). In a study of 26 obese women of varying adipose organ cellularity, Bjorntorp et al. (17) showed that failure to further reduce body weight on a hypocaloric diet occurred once normal fat cell size was achieved. These results are comparable to those in adult rats where hypercaloric, high fat diet-induced adipocyte hyperplasia is followed by a return to normal cell size (despite adipose organ hyperplasia) when the diet is restored to normal rat chow (55).

These findings have potential implications for the prevention and treatment of obesity. Inhibition of adipocyte synthesis, if possible, might prevent hyperplastic obesity due both to genetic and environmental influences. Such an achievement is clearly far beyond our current understanding of molecular biology in general and adipose organ development in particular. In treating obesity a distinction between types of patients with regard to cellularity and cell size would probably be helpful. The severely hyperplastic obese (who fortunately constitute only a small fraction of all obese patients) should perhaps not be expected to achieve a body composition as near normal as their less hyperplastic peers. Reduced expectations could relieve some of the psychological agony (for both patient and physician) attending efforts at controlling weight in this special subgroup. Clinical attention should be focused on adipocyte size as a predictor of potential for response to therapy and success at maintaining reduced weight. Efforts to reduce weight to a point where adipocyte size is "subnormal" will almost always fail in the long-term. The patient should be made to understand that total adipose mass is a product of cell size and number, that size can be readily reduced to a normal range, but that number cannot be diminished, and that, therefore, those with an excessive number of adipocytes can achieve a normal adipose mass only by reducing cell size below normal. Since there appear to be a variety of counterregulatory processes tending to return cell size to normal, patients usually have great difficulty in sustaining normal weight at the cost of subnormal adipocyte size.

CONCLUSIONS

The specific factors governing the development of the adipose organ in man and animals are incompletely understood. With the exception of certain inbred rodent strains, it is not yet possible to apportion conclusively the relative contributions of genotype and environment to the size of the adipose organ at any period of development. The following generalizations may be made with regard to human adipose tissue and obesity.

First, the apparent dichotomy between the "cell counting" and "energy metabolism defect" schools of obesity is a false one. (a) Regardless of how many adipocytes are formed, for whatever reason, they must be filled with lipid if obesity is to occur. Such filling can only occur when the individual is in net positive energy balance because of excessive calorie intake and/or a relative enhancement of metabolic efficiency. Obese patients do not have an absolute or relative deficit of lean body mass and, therefore, this filling of adipocytes is not simply a result of the "shunting" of calories away from lean tissue into fat. (b) Since cell size cannot enlarge beyond approximately 1.2 micrograms lipid/cell, moderate to severely obese individuals must have hyperplastic adipose tissue, clearly distinguishing them from less obese or normal individuals. This increased cell number may help to perpetuate obesity since therapeutic reduction of adipocyte size below "normal" is extremely difficult to achieve and maintain. Thus, abnormalities of *both* energy metabolism and adipose tissue geometry characterize the obese patient. The primary defect could reside in either the area of energy metabolism (including food intake) or adipocyte formation, or both. In different animal models and possibly in different types of human obesity, either cellular or energetic disturbances may be the primary event.

Second, the capacity for adipocyte formation probably remains present throughout life. Rates of formation at any period of life are dependent on both genetic and environmental influences, the former apparently predominating until early adulthood and the latter having relatively greater influence in later life. Achievement of a critical adipocyte volume may be the "signal" for hyperplasia in the adult. Infant feeding practices, although capable of producing transient changes in total adipose organ mass (possibly by accelerating the normal time course of development), probably do not exercise the sole or necessarily most significant influence on ultimate size of the adipose organ. The weak correlation between adiposity in infancy and early childhood probably reflects the early expression of genotype in some individuals destined to be obese rather than a causal relationship between early adiposity and later obesity.

Third, hyperplastic obesity is a real clinical entity and not the result of an artifact related to nonassayed visceral fat mass in nonobese or moderately obese individuals. There may be no correlation between age of onset of obesity and adipose organ cellularity, if the total weight of the adipose organ is factored out of the correlation. Hyperplastic obesity is much more rare than lesser degrees of obesity, and is difficult to treat successfully in the long term. This intractability, and the inverse relationship between cellularity and therapeutic success, may reflect persistence of environmental-behavioral influences that caused the obesity in the first place or the effects of homeostatic mechanisms tending to maintain a constant adipocyte volume regardless of adipocyte number, or the interaction of both factors.

Fourth, white adipocyte size may be maintained within a relatively narrow range by intrinsic biochemical processes as well as possible indirect effects on appetitive behavior. Although net substrate cycles within WAT are not sufficiently exothermic to contribute significantly to organismic thermogenesis, BAT has the specialized biochemical machinery to permit such a role. Although BAT plays a role in non-shivering thermogenesis in the human neonate, its role in adult man is unclear.

ACKNOWLEDGMENTS

Work on this chapter was supported in part by a grant from the NIH (5 RO1 AM 18325), and by a Public Health Service Fogarty International Research Fellowship to Dr. Berry (5 FO5 TWO2918–02). Dr. Leibel is a Rockefeller Scholar in clinical science. The authors gratefully acknowledge the expert secretarial assistance of Mrs. Virginia Rosario.

REFERENCES

1. Abumrad, N. A., Perkins, R. C., Park, J. H., and Park, C. R. (1981): Mechanism of long chain fatty acid permeation on the isolated adipocyte. *J. Biol. Chem.*, 256:9183–9191.
2. Ackerman, G. E., Smith, M. E., Mendelson, C. R., Macdonald, P. C., and Simpson, E. R. (1981): Aromatization of androstenedione by human adipose tissue stromal cells in monolayer culture. *J. Clin. Endocrinol. Metab.*, 53:412–417.
3. Adebonojo, F. O. (1975): Studies on human adipose cells in culture: Relation of cell size and cell multiplication to donor age. *Yale J. Biol. Med.*, 48:9–16.
4. Angel, A. (1970): Studies on the compartmentation of lipid in adipose cells. I: Subcellular distribution, composition, and transport of newly synthesized lipid liposomes. *J. Lipid Res.*, 11:420–432.
5. Arner, P., and Ostman, J. (1976): Changes in the adrenergic control and the rate of lipolysis of isolated human adipose tissue during fasting and after refeeding. *Acta Med. Scand.*, 200:273–279.
6. Arner, P., and Ostman, J. (1980): Importance of the cyclic AMP concentration for the rate of lipolysis in human adipose tissue. *Clin. Sci.*, 59:199–201.
7. Asher, P. (1966): Fat babies and fat children. The prognosis of obesity in the very young. *Arch. Dis. Child.*, 41:672–673.
8. Ashwell, M., and Garrow, J. S. (1973): Full and empty fat cells. *Lancet*, 2:1036–1037.
9. Ashwell, M. A., Priest, P., and Bondoux, M. (1975): Adipose tissue cellularity in obese women: Relation to age of onset of obesity. In: *Recent Advances in Obesity Research, I*, edited by A. N. Howard, pp. 74–77. Newman, London.
10. Bagdade, J. D., and Hirsch, J. (1966): Gestational and dietary influence on the lipid content of the infant buccal fat pad. *Proc. Soc. Exp. Biol. Med.*, 122:616–619.
11. Omitted in proof.

12. Biron, P., Mongeau, J. G., and Bertrand, D. (1977): Familial resemblance of body weight and weight/height in 374 homes with adopted children. *J. Pediatr.*, 91:555–558.
13. Bjorntorp, P. (1974): Effects of age, sex, and clinical conditions on adipose tissue cellularity in man. *Metabolism*, 23:1091–1102.
14. Bjorntorp, P. (1977): The fat cell: A clinical view. In: *Recent Advances in Obesity Research II: Proceedings of the 2nd International Congress on Obesity*, edited by G. Bray, pp. 153–168. Newman, London.
15. Bjorntorp, P. (1981): Adipocyte precursor cells. In: *Recent Advances in Obesity Research III*, edited by P. Bjorntorp, M. Cairella, and A. N. Howard. pp. 58–69. John Libbey, London.
16. Bjorntorp, P., Bengtsson, C., Blohme, G., Jansson, A., Sjostrom, L., Tibblin, E., Tibblin, G., and Wilhelmsen, L. (1971): Adipose tissue fat cell size and number in relation to metabolism in randomly selected middle-aged men and women. *Metabolism*, 20:927–935.
17. Bjorntorp, P., Carlgren, G., Isaksson, B., Kratkiewski, M., Larsson, B., and Sjostrom, L. (1975): Effect of and energy-reduced dietary requirements in relation to adipose tissue cellularity in obese women. *Am. J. Clin. Nutr.*, 28:445–452.
18. Bjorntorp, P., Karlsson, M., and Gustaffson, L. (1979): Quantitation of different cells in the epididymal fat pad of the rat. *J. Lipid Res.*, 20:97–106.
19. Bjorntorp, P., Karlsson, M., and Pertoft, H. (1978): The isolation and characterization of cells from rat adipose tissue developing into adipocytes. *J. Lipid Res.*, 19:316–324.
20. Bjorntorp, P., and Sjostrom, L. (1971): Number and size of adipose tissue fat cells in relation to metabolism in human obesity. *Metabolism*, 20:703–713.
21. Bjorntorp, P., and Sjostrom, L. (1979): Adipose tissue cellularity. *Int. J. Obes.*, 3:181–187.
22. Bjorntorp, P., and Vrana, J. (1971): Microscopic fat cell size measurement on frozen-cut adipose tissue in comparison with automatic determinations of osmium-fixed fat cells. *J. Lipid Res.*, 12:521–530.
23. Bjurulf, P. (1959): Atherosclerosis and body build with special reference to size and number of subcutaneous fat cells. *Acta Med. Scand.*, Suppl. 166:7–9.
24. Booth, D. A. (1980): Acquired behavior controlling energy intake and output. In: *Obesity*, edited by A. J. Stunkard, pp. 101–143. W. B. Saunders Company, Philadelphia.
25. Borjeson, M. (1976): The aetiology of obesity in children. *Acta Paediatr. Scand.*, 65:279–287.
26. Bray, G. A. (1976): *The Obese Patient*, pp. 44–93, 129–155. W. B. Saunders, Philadelphia.
27. Bray, G. A. (1981): The inheritance of corpulence. In: *The Body Weight Regulatory System: Normal and Disturbed Mechanisms*, edited by L. A. Cioffi, W. P. T. James, and T. Van Itallie, pp. 185–195. Raven Press, New York.
28. Brook, C. G. D. (1978): Cellular growth: Adipose tissue. In: *Human Growth, Vol. 2: Post Natal Growth*, edited by F. Faulkner and J. M. Tanner, pp. 21–33. Plenum Press, New York.
29. Brook, C. G. D., Huntley, R. M. C., and Slack, J. (1975): Influence of heredity and environment in determination of skinfold thickness in children. *Br. Med. J.*, 2:719–721.
30. Brook, C. G. D., Lloyd, J., and Wolff, O. H. (1972): Relationship between age of onset of obesity and size and number of adipose cells. *Br. Med. J.*, 2:25–27.
31. Burns, T. W., Boyer, P. A., Terry, B. F., Langley, P. E., and Robison, G. A. (1979): The effect of fasting on the adrenergic receptor activity of human adipocytes. *J. Lab. Clin. Med.*, 94:387–394.
32. Burns, T. W., Langley, P. E., Terry, B. E., Bylund, D. B., Hoffman, B. B., Tharp, M. D., Lefkowitz, R. J., Garcia-Sainz, A., and Fain, J. N. (1981): Pharmacologic characterizations of adrenergic receptors in human adipocytes. *J. Clin. Invest.*, 67:467–475.
33. Burns, T. W., Langley, P. E., Terry, B. E., and Robison, G. A. (1978): The role of free fatty acids in the regulation of lipolysis by human adipose tissue cells. *Metabolism*, 27:1755–1762.
34. Butcher, R. W. (1966): Cyclic 3'5' AMP and the lipolytic effects of hormones on adipose tissue. *Pharmacol. Rev.*, 18:237–241.
35. Butcher, R. W., Baird, C. E., and Sutherland, E. W. (1968): Effect of lipolytic and antilipolytic substances on adenosine 3'5' monophosphate in isolated fat cells. *J. Biol. Chem.*, 243:1705–1712.
36. Charney, E., Goodman, H. C., McBride, M., Lyon, B., and Pratt, R. (1976): Childhood antecedents of adult obesity. Do chubby infants become obese adults? *N. Engl. J. Med.*, 295:6–9.
37. Cheung, W. Y. (1980): Calmodulin plays a pivotal role in cellular regulation. *Science*, 207:19–27.
38. Chumlea, W. C., Knittle, J. L., Roche, A. F., Siervogel, R. M., and Webb, P. (1981): Size and number of adipocytes and measures of body fat in boys and girls 10 to 18 years of age. *Am. J. Clin. Nutr.*, 34:1791–1797.

39. Chumlea, W. C., Roche, A. F., Siervogel, R. M., Knittle, J. L., and Webb, P. (1981): Adipocytes and adiposity in adults. *Am. J. Clin. Nutr.*, 34:1798–1803.
40. Clarkson, P. M., Katch, F. I., Kroll, W., Lane, R., and Kamen, G. (1980): Regional adipose cellularity and reliability of adipose cell size determination. *Am. J. Clin. Nutr.*, 33:2245–2252.
41. Clarkson, P. M., Kroll, W., Wai, J., and Kamen, G. (1981): A comparison of four methods to measure fat cell size. *Am. J. Clin. Nutr.*, 34:2287–2290.
42. Comstock, G. W., and Stone, R. W. (1972): Changes in body weight and subcutaneous fat thickness related to smoking habits. *Arch. Environ. Health*, 24:271–276.
43. Daniel, H., and Derry, D. M. (1969): Criteria for differentiation of brown and white fat in the rat. *Can. J. Physiol. Pharmacol.*, 47:941–945.
44. Dauncey, M. J., and Gardner, D. (1975): Size of adipose cells in infancy. *Arch. Dis. Child.*, 50:286–290.
45. Dawkins, M., and Hull, D. (1965): The production of heat by fat. *Sci. Am.*, 213:62–67.
46. Derry, D. M., Schonbaum, E., and Steiner, G. (1969): Two sympathetic nerve supplies to brown adipose tissue of the rat. *Can. J. Physiol. Pharmacol.*, 47:57–63.
47. DeSwiet, M., Fayers, P., and Cooper, L. (1977): Effects of feeding habit on weight in infancy. *Lancet*, 1:892–894.
48. Dobbing, J. (1974): The later development of the brain and its vulnerability. In: *Scientific Foundations of Paediatrics*, edited by J. A. Davis and J. Dobbing, pp. 565–577. W. B. Saunders Co., Philadelphia.
49. Dubois, S., Hill, D. E., and Beaton, G. H. (1979): An examination of factors believed to be associated with infantile obesity. *Am. J. Clin. Nutr.*, 32:1997–2004.
50. Durnin, J. V. G. A., and Womersley, J. (1974): Body fat assessed from total body density and its estimation from skinfold thickness: Measurements on 481 men and women aged from 16 to 72 years. *Br. J. Nutr.*, 32:77–97.
51. Eid, E. E. (1970): Follow up study of physical growth of children who had excessive weight gain in the first six months of life. *Br. Med. J.*, 2:74–76.
52. Enzi, G., Zanardo, V., Caretta, F., Inelmen, E. M., and Rubaltelli, F. (1981): Intrauterine growth and adipose tissue development. *Am. J. Clin. Nutr.*, 34:1785–1790.
53. Fain, J. N., and Garcia-Sainz, J. A. (1980): Role of phosphatidylinositol turnover in alpha$_1$, and of adenylate cyclase inhibition in alpha$_2$ effects of catecholamines. *Life Sci.*, 26:1183–1194.
54. Faust, I. M. (1980): Nutrition and the fat cell. *Int. J. Obes.*, 4:314–321.
55. Faust, I. M., Johnson, P. R., Stern, J. S., and Hirsch, J. (1978): Diet-induced adipocyte number increase in adult rats: A new model of obesity. *Am. J. Physiol.*, 235:E279–E286.
56. Foch, T. T., and McClearn, G. E. (1980): Genetics, body weight, and obesity. In: *Obesity*, edited by A. J. Stunkard, pp. 48–71. W. B. Saunders Company, Philadelphia.
57. Forbes, G. B., and Reina, J. C. (1970): Adult lean body mass declines with age: Some longitudinal observations. *Metabolism*, 19:653–663.
58. Foster, D. O., and Frydman, M. L. (1979): Tissue distribution of cold-induced thermogenesis in conscious warm- or cold-acclimated rats re-evaluated from changes in tissue blood flow: The dominant role of brown adipose tissue in the replacement of shivering by nonshivering thermogenesis. *Can. J. Physiol. Pharmacol.*, 57:257–270.
59. Fredholm, B. B. (1978): Local regulation of lipolysis in adipose tissue by fatty acids, prostaglandins and adenosine. *Med. Biol.*, 56:249–261.
60. Frisch, R. E., and McArthur, J. W. (1974): Menstrual cycles: Fatness as a determinant of minimum weight for height necessary for their maintenance or onset. *Science*, 185:949–951.
61. Frisch, R. E., Wyshak, G., and Vincent, L. (1980): Delayed menarche and amenorrhea in ballet dancers. *N. Engl. J. Med.*, 303:17–19.
62. Garn, S. M., and Clark, D. C. (1976): Trends in fatness and the origins of obesity. *Pediatrics*, 57:443–456.
63. Giacobino, J. P., and Chmelar, M. (1977): Fatty acid esterification in adipocyte subcellular fractions. *Int. J. Biochem.*, 8:413–416.
64. Glick, Z., Teague, R. J., and Bray, G. A. (1981): Brown adipose tissue: Response increased by a single low protein, high carbohydrate meal. *Science*, 213:1125–1127.
65. Goldrick, R. B., and Galton, D. J. (1974): Fatty acid synthesis de novo in human adipose tissue. *Clin. Sci. Mol. Med.*, 46:469–479.
66. Goldrick, R. B., and McLaughlin, G. M. (1970): Lipolysis and lipogenesis from glucose in human fat cells of different sizes. *J. Clin. Invest.*, 49:1213–1223.

67. Goodman, D. B. (1958): The interaction of human serum albumin with long-chain fatty acid anions. *J. Am. Chem. Soc.*, 80:3892–3898.
68. Goodman, M. H. (1970): Permissive effects of hormones on lipolysis. *Endocrinology*, 86:1064–1074.
69. Gordon, R. S., and Cherkes, A. (1956): Unesterified fatty acid in human blood plasma. *J. Clin. Invest.*, 35:206–212.
70. Gordon, T., and Kannel, W. B. (1976): Obesity and cardiovascular disease: The Framingham Study. *Clin. Endocrinol. Metab.*, 5:367–375.
71. Green, H., and Kehinde, O. (1974): Subtypes of mouse 3T3 cells that accumulate lipid. *Cell*, 1:113–116.
72. Greenwood, M. R. C., and Hirsch, J. (1974): Postnatal development of adipocyte cellularity in the normal rat. *J. Lipid Res.*, 15:474–483.
73. Gurr, M. I., and Kirtland, J. (1978): Adipose tissue cellularity: A review 1. Techniques for studying cellularity. *Int. J. Obes.*, 2:401–427.
74. Hager, A. (1977): Adipose cell size and number in relation to obesity. *Postgrad. Med. J.*, 53:101–107.
75. Hager, A., Sjostrom, L., Arvidsson, B., Bjorntorp, P., and Smith, U. (1977): Body fat and adipose tissue cellularity in infants: A longitudinal study. *Metabolism*, 26:607–614.
76. Hager, A., Sjostrom, L., Arvidsson, B., Bjorntorp, P., and Smith, U. (1978): Adipose tissue cellularity in obese school girls before and after dietary treatment. *Am. J. Clin. Nutr.*, 31:68–75.
77. Hahn, P., and Novak, M. (1975): Development of brown and white adipose tissue. *J. Lipid Res.*, 16:79–91.
78. Hales, C. N., Luzio, J. P., and Siddle, K. (1978): Hormonal control of adipose tissue lipolysis. *Biochem. Soc. Symp.*, 43:97–135.
79. Heaton, G. M., and Nicholls, D. G. (1976): Hamster brown adipose tissue mitochondria. The role of fatty acids in the control of the proton conductance of the inner membrane. *Eur. J. Biochem.*, 67:511–517.
80. Heaton, J. M. (1972): The distribution of brown adipose tissue in the human. *J. Anat.*, 112:35–39.
81. Himms-Hagen, J. (1980): Current status of nonshivering thermogenesis. In: *Assessment of Energy Metabolism in Health and Disease*, Report of First Ross Conference on Medical Research, edited by J. Kinney, pp. 92–102. Ross Laboratories, Columbus, Ohio.
82. Himms-Hagen, J., and Desautels, M. (1978): A mitochondrial defect in brown adipose tissue of the obese (ob/ob) mouse: Reduced binding of purine nucleotides and a failure to respond to cold by an increase in binding. *Biochem. Biophys. Res. Commun.*, 83:628–634.
83. Hinkle, P. C., and McCarty, R. E. (1978): How cells make ATP. *Sci. Am.*, 238:104–123.
84. Hirsch, J., and Batchelor, B. (1976): Adipose tissue cellularity in human obesity. *Clin. Endocrinol. Metab.*, 5:299–311.
85. Hirsch, J., and Gallian, E. (1968): Methods for the determination of adipose cell size in man and animals. *J. Lipid Res.*, 9:110–118.
86. Horwitz, B. A. (1973): Ouabain-sensitive component of brown fat thermogenesis. *Am. J. Physiol.*, 224:352–355.
87. James, W. P. T., and Trayhurn, P. (1981): Thermogenesis and obesity. *Br. Med. Bull.*, 37:43–48.
88. Johnson, P. R., Stern, J. S., Greenwood, M. R. C., Zucker, L. M., and Hirsch, J. (1973): Effect of early nutrition on adipose cellularity and pancreatic insulin release in the Zucker rat. *J. Nutr.*, 103:738–743.
89. Jung, T., Gurr, M. F., Robinson, M. P., and James, W. P. T. (1978): Does adipocyte hypercellularity in obesity exist? *Br. Med. J.*, 2:319–321.
90. Jungas, R. L., and Ball, E. G. (1963): The effect of insulin and epinephrine on free fatty acid and glycerol production in the presence and absence of glucose. *Biochemistry*, 2:383–388.
91. Khoo, J. C., Aguino, A. A., and Steinberg, D. (1974): The mechanism of activation of hormone-sensitive lipase in human adipose tissue. *J. Clin. Invest.*, 53:1124–1131.
92. Khoo, J. C., Steinberg, D., Thompson, B., and Mayer, S. E. (1973): Hormonal regulation of adipocyte enzymes. *J. Biol. Chem.*, 248:3823–3830.
93. Kirtland, J., and Gurr, H. I. (1979): Adipose tissue cellularity: A review. 2. The relationship between cellularity and obesity. *Int. J. Obes.*, 3:15–55.
94. Kirtland, J., Gurr, M. I., Saville, G., and Widdowson, E. M. (1975): Occurrence of pockets of very small cells in adipose tissue of the guinea pig. *Nature*, 256:723–724.
95. Knittle, J. L. (1978): Adipose tissue development in man. In: *Human Growth, Vol. 2: Post Natal Growth*, edited by F. Faulkner and J. M. Tanner, pp. 295–315. Plenum Press, New York.

96. Knittle, J., and Hirsch, J. (1968): Effect of early nutrition on the development of rat epididymal fat pads: Cellularity and metabolism. *J. Clin. Invest.*, 47:2091–2098.
97. Knittle, J. L., Timmers, K., Ginsberg-Fellner, F., Brown, R. E., and Katz, D. P. (1979): The growth of adipose tissue in children and adolescents. *J. Clin. Invest.*, 63:239–246.
98. Koerker, D. J., Goodner, C. J., Chideckel, E. W., and Ensinck, J. W. (1975): Adaptation to fasting in baboon. II. Regulation of lipolysis early and late in fasting. *Am. J. Physiol.*, 229:350–354.
99. Krauss, R. M., Herbert, P. N., Levy, R. I., and Fredrickson, D. S. (1973): Further observations on the activities and inhibitions of lipoprotein lipase by apolipoproteins. *Circ. Res.*, 33:403–411.
100. Krotkiewski, M., Sjostrom, L., and Bjorntorp, P. (1977): Adipose tissue cellularity in relation to prognosis for weight reduction. *Int. J. Obes.*, 1:395–416.
101. Laurell, S. (1957): Turnover rate of unesterified fatty acids in human plasma. *Acta Physiol. Scand.*, 41:158–167.
102. Ledbetter, D. H., Riccardi, V. M., Airhart, S. D., Strobel, R. J., Kunan, B. S., and Crawford, J. D. (1981): Deletions of chromosome 15 as a cause of the Prader-Willi syndrome. *N. Engl. J. Med.*, 304:325–329.
103. Leibel, R. L. (1977): A biologic radar system for the assessment of body mass. The model of a geometry sensitive endocrine system is presented. *J. Theor. Biol.*, 66:297–306.
104. Leibel, R.L. (1981): Some aspects of energy metabolism relevant to obesity. In: *Human Nutrition: Clinical and Biochemical Aspects*, edited by P. J. Garry, 239–254. The American Association for Clinical Chemistry, Washington, D.C.
105. Lindberg, O., editor (1970): *Brown Adipose Tissue*. American Elsevier Publishing Company, Inc., New York.
106. Marshall, W. A. (1978): Puberty. In: *Human Growth 2. Postnatal Growth*, edited by F. Falkner and J. M. Tanner, pp. 141–181. Plenum Press, New York.
107. Mayer, S. E. (1980): Drugs acting at synaptic and neuroeffector junctional sites. In: *The Pharmacological Basis of Therapeutics, Sixth Edition*, edited by A. G. Gilman, L. S. Goodman, and A. Gilman, pp. 56–90. Macmillan, New York.
108. Melbin, T., and Vuille, J. C. (1973): Physical development at seven years of age in relation to velocity of weight gain in infancy with special reference to overweight. *Br. J. Prev. Soc. Med.*, 27:225–235.
109. Mitchell, P. (1979): Keilin's respiratory chain concept and its chemiosmotic consequences. *Science*, 206:1148–1159.
110. Mrosovsky, N., and Rowlatt, U. (1968): Changes in microstructure of brown fat at birth in the human infant. *Biol. Neonate*, 13:230–252.
111. Neumann, R. O. (1902): Experimentelle beitrage zur lehre von dem taglichen nahrungsbedarf des menschen unter besonderer berucesichtigung der notwendigen eiweifsmenge. *Arch. Hygeine*, 45:1–87. Cited by Bray, ref. 26, p. 154.
112. Newsholme, E. A., and Start, C. (1973): Adipose tissue and the regulation of fat metabolism. In: *Regulation in Metabolism*, pp. 216–217. John Wiley & Sons, London.
113. Nicholls, D. C. (1976): Hamster brown-adipose tissue mitochondria. Purine nucleotide control of the ion conductance of the inner membrane, the nature of the nucleotide binding site. *Eur. J. Biochem.*, 62:223–228.
114. Nimrod, A., and Ryan, K. (1975): Aromatization of androgens by human abdominal and breast fat tissue. *J. Clin. Endocrinol. Metab.*, 40:367–372.
115. Oschry, Y., and Shapiro, B. (1981): Fat associated with adipose lipase. The newly synthesized fraction that is the preferred substrate for lipolysis. *Biochim. Biophys. Acta*, 664:201–206.
116. Ostman, G., Arner, P., Engfeldt, P., and Kager, L. (1979): Regional differences in the control of lipolysis in human adipose tissue. *Metabolism*, 28:1198–1205.
117. Ostman, J., Backman, L., and Hallberg, D. (1973): Cell size and lipolysis by human subcutaneous adipose tissue. *Acta Med Scand.*, 193:969–975.
118. Owen, O. E., and Reichard, G. A. (1971): Fuels consumed by man: The interplay between carbohydrates and fatty acids. *Prog. Biochem. Pharmacol.*, 6:177–213.
119. Owen, O. E., Reichard, G. A., Jr., Boden, G., Patel, M. S., and Trapp, V. E. (1978): Interrelationships among key tissues in the utilization of metabolic substrates. In: *Advances in Modern Nutrition, Volume 2: Diabetes, Obesity and Vascular Disease*, edited by H. M. Katzen and R. J. Mahler, pp. 517–550. Hemisphere Publishing Co., Washington, D.C.
120. Pace, N., and Rathbun, E. N. (1945): Studies on body composition, body water and chemically combined nitrogen content in relation to fat content. *J. Biol. Chem.*, 158:685–691.

121. Patel, S. M., Owen, O. E., Goldman, L. I., and Hanson, R. W. (1975): Fatty acid synthesis by human adipose tissue. *Metabolism*, 24:161–173.
122. Patten, R. L. (1970): The reciprocal regulation of lipoprotein lipase activity and hormone-sensitive lipase activity in rat adipocytes. *J. Biol. Chem.*, 245:5577–5584.
123. Perkins, M. H., Rothwell, N. J., Stock, M. J., and Stone, T. W. (1981): Activation of brown adipose tissue thermogenesis by the ventromedial hypothalamus. *Nature*, 289:401–402.
124. Poskitt, E. M. E., and Cole, T. J. (1977): Do fat babies stay fat? *Br. Med. J.*, 1:7–9.
125. Pykalisto, O. J., Smith, P. H., and Brunzell, J. D. (1975): Determinants of human adipose tissue lipoprotein lipase. *J. Clin. Invest.*, 56:1108–1117.
126. Ravelli, G. P., Stein, Z. A., and Susser, M. W. (1976): Obesity in young men after famine exposure in utero and early infancy. *N. Engl. J. Med.*, 295:349–353.
127. Rodbell, M. (1965): Modulation of lipolysis in adipose tissue by free fatty acid concentrations in fat cells. *Ann. NY Acad. Sci.*, 131:302–314.
128. Roncari, D. A. K., and Van, R. L. R. (1978): Promotion of human adipocyte precursor replication of 17, beta estradiol in culture. *J. Clin. Invest.*, 62:503–508.
129. Rosenquist, U. (1972): Inhibition of noradrenaline-induced lipolysis in hypothyroid subjects by increased alpha-adrenergic responsiveness. *Acta Med. Scand.*, 192:353–359.
130. Rothwell, N. J., and Stock, M. J. (1979): A role for brown adipose tissue in diet-induced thermogenesis. *Nature*, 281:31–35.
131. Salans, L. B., Cushman, S. W., and Weisman, R. E. (1973): Studies of human adipose tissue: Adipose cell size and number in non-obese and obese patients. *J. Clin. Invest.*, 52:929–941.
132. Salans, L. B., Horton, E. S., and Sims, E. A. H. (1971): Experimental obesity in man. *J. Clin. Invest.*, 50:1005–1011.
133. Scow, R. O., Blanchette-Mackie, E. J., and Smith, L. C. (1976): Role of capillary endothelium in the clearance of chylomicrons. *Circ. Res.*, 39:149–162.
134. Scow, R. O., Hamosh, M., Blanchette Mackie, E. J., and Avans, A. J. (1972): Uptake of blood triglycerides by various tissue. *Lipids*, 7:495–505.
135. Shapiro, B. (1977): Adipose tissue. In: *Lipid Metabolism in Mammals*, edited by F. Snyder, pp. 287–316. Plenum Press, New York.
136. Shimazu, T., and Takahashi, A. (1980): Stimulation of hypothalamic nuclei has differential effects on lipid synthesis in brown and white adipose tissue. *Nature*, 284:62–63.
137. Sims, E. A. (1976): Experimental obesity, dietary induced thermogenesis, and their clinical implications. *Clin. Endocrinol. Metab.*, 5:377–395.
138. Sjostrom, L. (1980): Fat cells and body weight. In: *Obesity*, edited by A. J. Stunkard, pp. 72–100. W. B. Saunders Company, Philadelphia.
139. Sjostrom, L., and Bjorntorp, P. (1974): Body composition and adipose tissue cellularity in human obesity. *Acta Med. Scand.*, 195:201–211.
140. Sjostrom, L., Bjorntorp, P., and Vrana, J. (1971): Microscopic cell size measurements on frozen-cut adipose tissue in comparison with automatic determinations of osmium-fixed fat cells. *J. Lipid Res.*, 12:521–530.
141. Sjostrom, L., Smith, U., Krotkiewski, M., and Bjorntorp, P. (1972): Cellularity in different regions of adipose tissue in young men and women. *Metabolism*, 21:1143–1153.
142. Smith, U. (1980): Adrenergic control of human adipose tissue lipolysis. *Eur. J. Clin. Invest.*, 10:343–344.
143. Smith, U., Hammersten, J., Bjorntorp, P., and Kral, J. (1979): Regional differences and effect of weight reduction on human fat cell metabolism. *Eur. J. Clin. Invest.*, 9:327–332.
144. Sorbris, R., Nilsson-Ehle, P., Monti, M., and Wadso, I. (1979): Differences in heat production between adipocytes from obese and normal weight individuals. *FEBS Lett.*, 101:411–414.
145. *Statistical Bulletin of the Metropolitan Life Insurance Co.* (1959): 40:1–4.
146. Stern, M. P., and Conrad, F. (1975): An automated, direct method for measuring adipocyte cell size. *Clin. Chim. Acta*, 65:29–37.
147. Suter, E. R. (1969): The fine structure of brown adipose tissue. I. Cold induced changes in the rat. *J. Ultrastruct. Res.*, 26:216–241.
148. Tanner, J. M. (1962): *Growth and Adolescence.* Blackwell Scientific Publications, Oxford.
149. Tanuma, Y., Ohata, M., Ito, T., and Yokochi, C. (1976). Possible function of human brown adipose tissue as suggested by observation on perirenal brown fats from necropsy cases of variable age groups. *Arch. Histol. Jpn.*, 39:117–145.
150. Tanuma, Y., Yamamoto, M., Ito, T., and Yokochi, C. (1975): The occurrence of brown adipose tissue in perirenal fat in Japanese. *Arch. Histol. Jpn.*, 38:43–70.

151. *Ten State Nutrition Survey 1968–1970* (1972): D.H.E.W. Publication No (H. S. M.) 72–8131.
152. Vague, J., and Fenasse, R. (1965): Comparative anatomy of adipose tissue. In: *Handbook of Physiology, Section 5: Adipose Tissue*, edited by A. E. Renold and G. F. Cahill, Jr., pp. 25–36. American Physiological Society, Washington, D.C.
153. Van, R. L. R., Bayliss, C. E., and Roncari, D. A. K. (1976): Cytological and enzymological characterization of adult human adipocyte precursors in culture. *J. Clin. Invest.*, 58:699–704.
154. Vaughan, M. (1962): The production and release of glycerol by adipose tissue incubated in vitro. *J. Biol. Chem.*, 237:3354–3358.
155. Widdowson, E. M., and Shaw, W. T. (1973): Full and empty fat cells. *Lancet*, 2:905.
156. Wilson, R. S. (1979): Analysis of longitudinal twin data. Basic model and applications to physical growth measures. *Acta Genet. Med. Gemellol. (Roma)*, 28:93–105.
157. Wilkinson, P. W., and Parkin, J. M. (1974): Fat cells in childhood obesity. *Lancet*, 2:1522.
158. Winick, M., and Noble, A. (1966): Cellular response in rats during malnutrition at various ages. *J. Nutr.*, 89:300–306.
159. Winick, M., and Noble, A. (1967): Cellular response with increased feeding in neonatal rats. *J. Nutr.*, 91:179–182.
160. Zierler, K. L. (1977): Fatty acids as substrates for heart and skeletal muscle. *Circ. Res.*, 54:35–39.
161. Zinder, O., Eisenberg, E., and Shapiro, B. (1973): Compartmentation of glycerides in adipose tissue cells. I. The mechanism of free fatty acid release. *J. Biol. Chem.*, 248:7673–7676.

Health and Obesity, edited by H. L. Conn, Jr.,
E. A. DeFelice, and P. Kuo. Raven Press,
New York © 1983.

Some Determinants of Body Fat Content

Theodore B. Van Itallie

*St. Lukes Medical Service, St. Luke's-Roosevelt Hospital Center and
the Department of Medicine and Institute of Human Nutrition,
Columbia University, College of Physicians and Surgeons, New York, New York 10025*

At the most superficial level, obesity appears to be a simple problem; however, the more we attempt to understand it, the more complex and elusive it becomes. This is because a host of different factors influence both sides of the energy balance equation—intake and expenditure. In addition, obesity is not a morphologically distinct entity; fat can be stored in a variety of distributions and in adipose depots that may be characterized by cellular enlargement, hyperplasia, or a mixture of both. A further complication is that some degree of "obesity" may be biologically desirable. The amount of fat that must be stored to ensure survival depends on the particular biological circumstances. For example, birds must store extra fat before they migrate over water, otherwise they could not make it because of lack of fuel (50). Similarly, bears need extra fat to get them through their winter sleep (26).

The point at which man's inventory of stored calories becomes a matter of clinical concern is not clearly demarcated. Unlike blood sugar, which is tightly regulated, the body's content of depot fat may vary widely to meet both biological and lifestyle needs. Also, as in one form of obesity, the amount of fat in the body simply may reflect an individual's inability to resist forces in the environment that strongly favor a high level of fat storage.

Thus, our understanding of obesity is as incomplete as our understanding of monetary inflation. Both phenomena are readily apparent but the underlying dynamics are often obscure.

To begin to understand obesity, we have to recognize that it results from the interplay of many factors. Although some of these factors have been tentatively identified, it is not possible at present to determine just how much each contributes to the final result, namely, the proportion of fat in the body at any given time. Also, the relative importance of the factors varies over time and from individual to individual.

In order to put the subject into better perspective, it is helpful to recall some of the many factors that are thought to be involved in the pathogenesis of human obesity. They are listed in Table 1. This list is not complete nor does it avoid some redundancy. But, to use the terminology of systems analysis, consideration of these elements will provide a sense of the multiplicity and variety of inputs that affect

TABLE 1. *Possible and likely determinants of human obesity*

Genetic
    Adipose tissue lipophilia (p)
    Impairment of nonshivering and/or diet-induced thermogenesis (p)
    Adipose tissue hyperplasia (l)
    Relatively low resting metabolic rate (l)
    Lack of athletic capability (p)
    Imbalance of hunger and satiety-related neuronal systems (p)
Environmental
    Diet composition (high in fat and sugar; low in starch and fiber) (l)
    Ready availability of a variety of palatable, calorically dense foods (l)
    Sedentary life-style (l)
    Excess use of alcoholic drinks (l)
    Frequent snacking (l)
    Occupation (p)
    Emotional factors (l)
Life cycle events
    Pregnancy (l)
    Aging (l)

p: possible; l: likely.

the particular output of the human homeostat that is under consideration—the size of the fat depot. From this examination, one can also obtain a notion of the kinds of things that must be changed if obesity is to be prevented or successfully treated.

DETERMINANTS OF BODY FAT CONTENT

In order to survive, the body requires energy on a continuing basis; therefore, it is not surprising that animals have evolved an elaborate system to ensure that fuel is always available. Once the umbilical cord is severed, we must rely entirely on our own reserves of energy and we must protect these reserves by replenishing them whenever possible. This we accomplish by seeking and ingesting food.

Physical Activity

In man, the size of the energy store, namely, the quantity of depot fat, is partly determined by life-style. Thus, the body fat content of the marathon runner is 5 to 10% of total weight (38) whereas that of the sumo wrestler may exceed 25% (35). In each case, body fat content is appropriate to the needs of the particular individual. The marathon runner cannot compete successfully if he is forced to carry a greater burden of fat than his competitor. In contrast, the sumo wrestler needs extra weight to make it possible to lean more heavily on his opponent.

Domestic animals generally maintain larger fat stores than do their feral counterparts (46). In the wild, carnivorous animals usually expend a great deal of energy in the search for food, food for which they must often compete. If it reduces agility and endurance and makes an animal more vulnerable to predators, excess body fat can be a fatal handicap.

Biological Imperatives

In the examples given thus far, it can be seen that in many instances the fat content of the body is strongly influenced by the physical activity level. This is partly true, but the situation is much more complex. There is evidence that some animals actively regulate body fat content in order to meet specific biological or phylogenetic needs. For example, hibernating animals increase fat stores prior to hibernation (50) and, during pregnancy, some animals accumulate extra fat in apparent anticipation of special postpartum needs (32).

Although the inventory of stored energy maintained by an animal can be biologically precious, other priorities such as the requirement to be highly mobile might override the animal's innate disposition to expand its fat depot. In other words, it is "adaptive" to have a good supply of stored energy but, in certain environmental circumstances, it is also "adaptive" to remain lean enough to be swift and agile. In such a situation the size of the fat depot would have to reflect a reconciliation of these two adaptational needs. If this is indeed the case, it becomes easier to rationalize the apparently inefficient use of food-derived energy by various mammals ranging from rat to man. By "inefficient" is meant the dissipation of an appreciable fraction of such energy as heat rather than its storage as fat. It appears that by the process of diet-induced thermogenesis (which will be discussed in more detail later) animals can partly protect themselves from the fattening effect of eating to excess.

Diet-Induced Thermogenesis and Nutriture

The ability that animals and humans have to waste energy after a meal may serve more than one useful purpose (46). True, this mechanism might help the animal avoid biologically unwanted obesity; however, it must be remembered that food provides more than calories. The ability to waste energy can help the animal obtain a more adequate supply of amino acids and other essential nutrients without incurring the hazard of becoming fat. This capability is important when the quality of the diet is suboptimal, for example, when the diet is low in protein content.

In recent years it has been observed that obese animals and humans eat less and lose weight on monotonous, relatively unpalatable diets (13,17), whereas lean animals and people eat more and gain weight when they are shifted from a tediously uniform diet to one that provides a variety of appetizing foods (39,40,48). Further investigation of this phenomenon has confirmed the previously untested assumption that satiety is sensory specific, and that animals and people will become satiated on one food but will retain appetite for another and yet another, different food (41).

When one reflects on the meaning of sensory-specific satiety, the admonition of nutritionists, "Eat a variety of foods," comes quickly to mind. To remain healthy (indeed, in order to survive), animals of all species must obtain an array of essential nutrients from their diets. In general, such an array is best provided by a variety of foods; hence the predilection for a varied, as opposed to a uniform, diet has survival value for some species. This bias in favor of variety becomes evident when certain strains of caged laboratory rats are placed on a "cafeteria" diet. In this kind of feeding situation the animals eat much more than usual and greatly increase their body fat content.

Diet Composition

Apart from its variety, the nature of the diet appears to influence body fat content. Thus, strict vegetarians (vegans) are slender (10,47), and obesity is rife among omnivorous Americans (1). Interestingly, long-term prospective studies of changes in body composition do not appear to have been reported in individuals systematically shifted from an omnivorous to a strictly vegetarian diet and vice versa.

IS BODY FAT CONTENT REGULATED?

From the foregoing comments, it should be clear that the body fat content in man and in most other mammals is significantly affected by such factors as level of physical activity, diet palatability and variety, nature of the diet, and the efficiency with which food energy is utilized. Other factors that have not been mentioned thus far such as aging and genetic makeup also influence the size of the fat depot. However, perhaps enough has been said to refute the notion that body fat, like blood sugar, is regulated independently of conditions in the environment. Yet, in spite of this manipulability of body fat content, the depot fat does seem to have considerable stability and is clearly under some form of regulation (57). For example, it is well recognized that when certain animals and human subjects are chronically depleted of their energy stores, they will spontaneously increase food intake and may also decrease energy expenditure so as to repair the deficit. Similarly, after neurologically intact animals have been rendered obese by force-feeding or induced to overeat by brain stimulation or insulin injections, they will spontaneously reduce food intake until energy stores return to or near the level observed in control animals. Finally, there is abundant evidence that, in the absence of illness or experimental manipulation, physically active nonobese animals and human subjects tend to maintain a relatively constant body weight for prolonged periods despite substantial fluctuations in energy expenditure. As Mrosovsky (32) has pointed out: "The assumption that levels of fat are regulated is not the same as the assumption that (the) regulatory systems are all powerful."

In the discussion to follow, several major components of the system that regulates the body's store of energy will be considered, first in sequence and then in relation to several integrative hypotheses. In this way, a few of the phenomena described above can be probed more deeply.

Because of its central role in the operation of the system under consideration, let us start by examining the role of the brain in the control of feeding behavior.

Role of Brain in Food Intake Control

It is more than 40 years since Hetherington and Ranson (18) reported their classic studies showing that experimentally induced bilateral damage in the ventromedial hypothalamus produces obesity in the rat. Subsequently, Brobeck et al. (3) demonstrated that the obesity so produced results largely from hyperphagia, and, a few years later, Anand and Brobeck (2) reported that bilateral damage in the extreme lateral portion of the hypothalamus results in aphagia.

These observations, together with studies of the effects of electrical stimulation of subareas of the hypothalamus, resulted in what is known as the "dual center" theory (53). This theory postulated that two principal subareas within the tuberal hypothalamus were involved in the central control of food intake. One of these subareas, the lateral hypothalamus (LH) was conceived of as being a "feeding center." This center was considered to be under the inhibitory influence of the other subarea, the ventromedial hypothalamus (VMH), which was thought to to function as a "satiety center".

In recent years, however, evidence has been accumulating that is not compatible with many aspects of the dual center theory. It seems unlikely that the VMH and LH actually play specific roles in the control of ingestive behavior; moreover, the evidence is tenuous that the VMH normally exerts its inhibitory effects by acting directly on the lateral hypothalamic area. Thus, in light of more recent evidence (57), the dual center theory has been modified by the concept that diffuse excitatory and inhibitory neuronal systems controlling feeding course through the limbic system and the whole brain.

Monoamine-Specific Neuronal Pathways

Apart from such manipulations as electrical and chemostimulation of brain sites, electrolytic and biochemical lesions, discrete knife-cut transections, and electrical recordings from single neurons and neuronal populations, the introduction of histofluorescence methods into neuroanatomy has greatly enhanced our knowledge of many brain functions. For example, many of the feeding disorders induced by brain insult were initially believed to result from damage to specific hypothalamic structures. It is becoming increasingly clear that some of these disturbances in feeding behavior result from damage to monoamine-specific neural pathways that originate from cell bodies located in the brainstem. The identification of several of these pathways a little more than 20 years ago was made possible by use of a technique by which catecholamines and related compounds are rendered fluorescent when they are condensed with formaldehyde (11).

The results of some of these methods for studying brain function in relation to food intake control are summarized in Fig. 1.

The recognition that monoamine-specific pathways are involved in the control of eating behavior has made it easier to understand the actions of certain drugs that affect appetite (14). For example, in light of current knowledge about the monoamine-specific neuronal systems that are concerned with hunger and satiety, one would expect noradrenergic (amphetamine or diethylpropion) and serotonergic (fenfluramine) drugs to induce satiety, and antagonists to norepinephrine (chlorpromazine) and serotonin (cyproheptadine) to promote hunger.

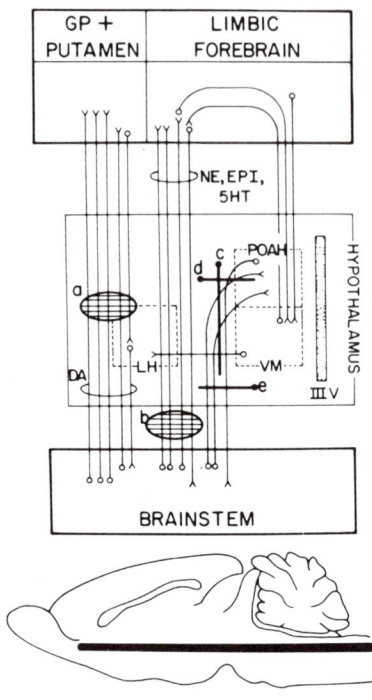

FIG. 1. Diagram of a near-horizontal section of the left half of the rat brain at the level shown by the inset **(bottom)**, indicating some of the possible feeding-related pathways disclosed by various types of neurological insult. Damage (indicated by hatched oval) to ascending dopamine (DA)-containing neurons **(a)** produces many of the ingestive abnormalities characteristically seen after ablation of the lateral hypothalamus (LH). Alterations in feeding behavior have also been produced by damage **(b)** to ascending noradrenergic (NE) and possibly adrenergic (EPI) and serotonergic (5HT) neurons, which may terminate near or project through the hypothalamus from the midbrain. Most of the components of the classic hypothalamic hyperphagia syndrome resulting from lesion damage in the vicinity of the ventromedial nucleus (VM) can also be effected by discrete knife cuts just lateral **(c)**, anterior **(d)**, or posterior **(e)** to this structure. The feeding effects produced by these neural transections and VM lesions appear to differ in many respects from those observed after selective destruction of neurochemically specific pathways. It is likely that some information related to feeding is also carried by reciprocating neural pathways between the limbic forebrain and the hypothalamus, and possibly between subareas within the hypothalamus. Other abbreviations: GP, globus pallidus; POAH, preoptic anterior hypothalamic region; III V, third ventricle. (From ref. 57 with permission.)

Interaction of "Feeding" and "Satiety" Systems

How then do the feeding and satiety systems actually influence eating behavior? Of course, no one knows for certain, but evidence is accumulating that there are "food reward" neurons in the LH that are responsive to certain sensory attributes of food such as sight, taste, and odor (42,43). The activity of these neurons is modulated by other neurons that are under the control of a variety of enteroceptive signals, such as gastric distention, gut hormone release, and glucose utilization, that collectively indicate whether or not the animal has eaten enough. Thus, by providing food reward to the hungry animal, food-related sensory inputs may normally elicit, direct, and maintain food ingestion. As the meal proceeds, the response of the food reward neurons to the sensory effects of the diet is altered by the buildup of stimuli signaling replenishment. In due course, eating is no longer pleasurable and, when food ceases to be rewarding, eating normally stops (20).

Up to this point, a picture of food intake control has been sketched out in which the balance of monoamine-specific neuronal systems concerned with feeding and satiety at any given time is thought to determine whether an animal will look for and ingest food, or whether it will be indifferent to food. Not yet indicated in any detail is the nature of the stimuli that signal satiety nor the ways in which such stimuli reach feeding-satiety neurons. Nor has any indication been given as to how the brain adjusts food intake so as to regulate the body's fat content. Let us briefly examine these aspects.

Satiety Signals

Obviously, an enormous amount of investigative work has been carried out in the attempt to throw more light on the phenomenon of satiety. No one signal has been identified that can induce and sustain satiety. In the past, it was thought that changes in blood glucose level or in the rate of glucose utilization might serve to tell the brain whether the body should be looking for food or whether, at that time, none was needed (56). Subsequent studies, however, showed that although glucose utilization rates often vary with meal-taking, one cannot predictably induce satiety by giving glucose intravenously, with or without added insulin (59). Actually, the evidence is quite good that the satiety signals that bring about cessation of eating originate in the upper gastrointestinal tract in response to food ingestion (52). As suggested earlier, such signals include those generated by the presence of food in the stomach (7,8) and by the arrival of gastric chyme in the duodenum and jejunum (25,28,29). Some of the signals may be transmitted via the vagus nerve from stretch receptors located in the stomach and small intestine (36). In addition, chemo-receptors in the stomach and upper small intestine may respond to food or to the products of digestion by releasing humoral substances capable of signaling satiety (58). Although it is assumed that the brain contains satiety receptors capable of detecting and responding to humoral agents arising from the gut, neither the nature nor the location of the putative receptors is known. Efforts have been made to demonstrate selective uptake by the hypothalamus of certain radioisotope-labeled hormones (such as insulin) and metabolites (such as glucose or glycerol) that might play a role in satiety. In a typical experiment the substance to be studied is injected intravenously into a rat and then some minutes later the brain of the animal is removed and radioautographs obtained from representative sections. Unfortunately, this technique has not yet been able to provide evidence for the existence of insulin-sensitive glucose receptors in the ventromedial hypothalamus (9). Nevertheless, this general approach is a promising one for the study of satiety-related events occurring in the brain.

Cholecystokinin and Other Gut Hormones

If it were possible to identify one or more humoral substances that normally contribute to satiety, then this information might be useful in the control of appetite in obese persons seeking to reduce their weight. A beginning has been made in this direction with the gut hormone cholecystokinin octapeptide, or CCK-8. Some workers believe that this peptide plays an important role in satiety (51). When CCK-8 is given intravenously to either nonobese or obese men, it can reduce meal size significantly; however, the effect is a small one (23)

ADAPTIVE THERMOGENESIS

We are accustomed to thinking about energy balance in terms of three major variables—the energy taken into the body as food, the energy expended in the form of basal or resting metabolism, and the energy expended as physical activity. It is commonly believed that physically active animals (including man) regulate body fat content by spontaneously increasing intake of dietary calories to compensate for an increased energy output. However, as animals and humans become more and more sedentary, their intake of food is not necessarily reduced to a corresponding degree, and body stores of fat may enlarge. In the sedentary range of activity, the nature, palatability, and variety of the habitual diet may play an increasingly important role in determining the body's fat content; thus, the caged rat may remain relatively lean on a low-fat diet that provides little or no variety. But, as we have seen, when the rat's diet is changed to one composed of foods obtained from the supermarket, body fat stores may enlarge.

With regard to the energy balance equation, increasing attention has been paid in recent years to the phenomenon of adaptive thermogenesis and its possible role in protecting animals against excess fat storage. It will be recalled that at the turn of the century, Neuman (33) reported that his weight remained relatively constant even though he systematically made substantial increases in his energy intake. This experience led him to coin the term "luxus konsumption," to describe the ability of the body to burn off excess energy when overfeeding occurs.

In relation to the problem of obesity, the question arises as to whether luxus konsumption protects some people against excess fat storage and impairment of the putative luxus konsumption mechanism renders others vulnerable to obesity. The picture in man is a confused one, but it may be helpful, first of all, to look at some of the information generated recently in animal experiments.

Gurr et al. (16) found that if they maintained weight in one group of weanling pigs by protein restriction and in another group by energy restriction, it could be shown that the protein-restricted animals had to take in three times as much energy to maintain weight as did the group whose protein intake was adequate. It was concluded that the extra calorie requirement for weight maintenance in the protein-restricted hyperphagic pigs was due mainly to diet-induced thermogenesis (DIT). Similar effects of protein restriction have been reported in weanling and adult rats (27,30).

Diet-Induced Thermogenesis and Brown Adipose Tissue

Recent studies reported by Stock and Rothwell (54) have provided information about DIT in rodents that may be relevant to human obesity. They induced hyperphagia and obesity in rats by offering them a cafeteria or snack-food diet of the type developed by Scalfani and Springer (48). In this case, the rats received their stock diet plus four palatable foods, e.g., cakes, popcorn, chocolate, and ham. Each day the choice of these four palatable foods was changed. On this diet, the energy intake of the rats was increased by more than 80%. However, it was evident that, although the rats gained weight and took on an obese appearance, the efficiency with which they were using the excess calories from the cafeteria diet was relatively low. When the brown adipose tissue (BAT) of these rats was examined, it was found to be substantially enlarged over that observed in controls. Moreover, it was demonstrated that, in the cafeteria rats, the contribution made by BAT to the thermogenic response to infused norepinephrine was much greater than that of control animals.

Intraspecies Differences in Efficiency of Energy Use

It was of interest that, although rats of the same strain (Sprague-Dawley) and age (75 days) had been used for all of these studies, the degree of obesity attained by rats maintained in two separate colonies differed markedly. Although both groups had increased food intake to the same extent (80%) when fed the cafeteria diet, the rats from one colony (A) gained 2.2 times more weight than their controls, whereas the rats from the other colony (B) gained only 1.5 times more weight than their controls. The greater body weight and energy gain of the rats in Colony A was shown by the authors to be due to a smaller energy output (2,740 versus 3,110 kJ) over the 8-day experiment. Rothwell and Stock (44) have suggested that subtle intrastrain differences in genotype can profoundly influence the metabolic response to hyperphagia. Because they represent a genetically heterogeneous population, human beings would be expected to show even greater variations in metabolic response to an increased food intake.

As pointed out by Rothwell and Stock (45), without the adaptive changes in DIT, the energy gain of cafeteria-fed rats would have been twice as great in Colony A and 5 times greater in Colony B.

Similarities Between Thermoregulatory and DIT

The mechanism of DIT has been the subject of considerable investigation. It has been customary to divide thermogenesis into two major categories, DIT and non-shivering or thermoregulatory thermogenesis (NST). Many similarities have been demonstrated between NST and DIT. Cold-adapted rats and rats that have gained weight on cafeteria-type diets show improved tolerance to cold, increased metabolic rates that are reduced by beta-adrenergic blockage, increased norepinephrine turnover, and enhanced thermogenic and lipolytic responses to norepinephrine (54).

Catecholamine Stimulation of BAT

It has been known for some time that BAT is an important source of heat production in hibernators and cold-adapted animals (19). Foster and Frydman (12) have used radioactively labeled microspheres to show that there is an extraordinarily high rate of blood flow and enhanced metabolic activity in the BAT of adult rats when they are either injected with norepinephrine (NE) or acutely exposed to the cold. Chronic cold adaptation produces an even greater flow of blood to BAT and further augments the thermogenic response to NE.

Rothwell and Stock (45) have recently used the blood flow method of Foster and Frydman to estimate the contribution of BAT to DIT in rats gaining weight on a cafeteria diet. As indicated earlier, such animals show hypertrophy and hyperplasia of BAT. In the studies of Rothwell and Stock, NE infusion produced substantial increases in oxygen consumption of 2.4 and 5.0 ml O_2/min in control and cafeteria rats, respectively. The rise in BAT oxygen consumption was 1.01 ml/min in the control animals and 3.86 ml/min in the cafeteria group. Thus, all of the enhanced thermogenic response to NE appeared to be due to BAT.

On the basis of current information, it seems that NST and DIT operate via similar mechanisms, both involving sympathetic activation of BAT. In this regard, it is interesting to note that Landsberg and Young (24) have reported that overfeeding stimulates, and caloric restriction reduces, NE turnover in pancreas and liver.

Perkins et al. (37) have recently demonstrated that electrical stimulation of the VMH produces a large increase in temperature in the interscapular BAT. This effect is inhibited by beta-adrenergic blockade. This observation suggests that neuronal structures within or traversing the VMH can influence thermogenesis as well as food intake. On the basis of this preliminary finding, one can speculate that certain VMH lesions are capable of diminishing or eliminating sympathetic activation of BAT, thereby increasing the efficiency with which dietary energy can be stored as fat.

Reduced Thermogenic Capability and Obesity

In view of the finding that cafeteria-fed rats exhibit varying degrees of thermogenesis with corresponding variations in rate of depot fat accumulation, it is of particular interest that several animal models of obesity exhibit subnormal thermogenesis. The most dramatic example of this defect is the propensity of ob/ob obese mice (and obese Zucker rats) to die of hypothermia in a cold environmental temperature at which normal controls can maintain thermal homeostasis (21).

The evidence is compelling that the reduced thermogenesis shown by the ob/ob mouse is an important contributor to the marked obesity that characterizes this mutant (21). For example, Thurlby and Trayhurn (55) have used Foster and Frydman's (12) method to measure blood flow to the BAT of obese ob/ob mice. Compared to controls, the obese mutants show a diminished thermogenic response to NE injection and, on the basis of the results of a variety of experiments, James et al. (22) have concluded that depressed BAT activity accounts for the difference in the metabolic response to NE between lean and ob/ob mice.

Mechanism of BAT Thermogenesis

At this juncture, it is appropriate to examine more closely the mechanism by which BAT can generate extra heat so effectively. In small rodents, most of the BAT is situated on the interscapular area and it comprises 1 to 2% of body weight. This tissue has a rich vasculature and it is heavily innervated with sympathetic fibers. As mentioned earlier, there is evidence for a direct neural link between the BAT and the VMH.

Research conducted by Nicholls (34) has provided the best available explanation of how BAT produces heat and this mechanism is shown in Fig. 2. The process of thermogenesis is apparently initiated by the release of NE at the nerve endings that penetrate the BAT. The NE binds to B_1-receptors on the surfaces of the cells of which BAT is composed. Such binding initiates a series of events that culminate in the hydrolysis of intracellular triglycerides, with the release of fatty acids and glycerol. In the course of their breakdown to acetyl-coenzyme A, the fatty acids release protons (hydrogen ions) that pass across the inner mitochondrial membrane. In other tissues, the transport of protons back through the membrane is normally associated with ATP synthesis. But in BAT, there exists a unique "proton conductance pathway" that permits protons to leak back into the mitochondrion without generating ATP. Thus, ATP synthesis is bypassed and heat is generated instead.

Not surprisingly, many workers in the field have hypothesized that at least some forms of human obesity may arise from impaired function of BAT. Studies are going on to test this hypothesis (5) but it is too early to make a firm prediction about the outcome of this work (15).

Thyroid Hormone Changes in Response to Over- and Underfeeding

Whenever metabolic rate is considered, it is inevitable that the status of the thyroid hormones will be examined. In this regard, Danforth and associates (6) have demonstrated that overfeeding is associated with increased concentrations in serum of T_3 and no change in the concentrations of T_4. At the same time, the production and metabolic clearance rate of T_3 are increased and the production and metabolic clearance rate of T_4 remain unchanged. When the intake of calories is at or below the level needed for weight maintenance, carbohydrate plays an important role in determining the concentrations of T_3 in the serum. When the car-

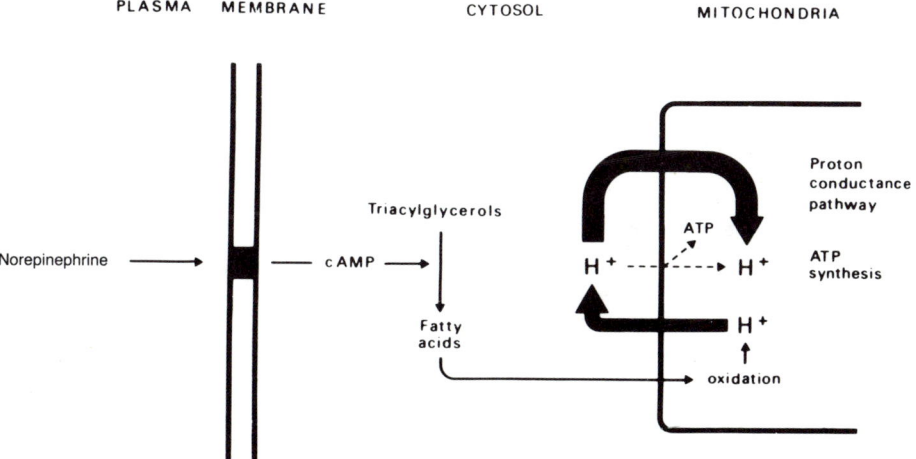

FIG. 2. Mechanism of thermogenesis in brown adipose tissue. From Trayhurn and James, ref. 55a, with permission.

bohydrate content of a eucaloric diet is reduced to very low levels, the mean concentration of serum T_3 falls significantly. As mentioned earlier, catecholamines are increased during overfeeding and decreased during underfeeding. Conceivably, the increased production and clearance of T_3 during overfeeding, in combination with an increased secretion of NE, might be responsible for the adaptive thermogenesis noted in nonobese and some obese subjects.

It has been hypothesized that some obese subjects are resistant to thyroid hormone action. A recent report (4) has appeared describing decreased concentrations of receptors for T_4 and T_3 in solubilized nuclei of circulating mononuclear cells from obese as compared with those from nonobese subjects. After weight reduction, the receptors from obese subjects still failed to respond normally. This preliminary observation suggests that further research is needed on larger numbers of lean and obese subjects in order to unravel further the possible role of adaptive thermogenesis in protecting individuals from excessive fat storage.

From the foregoing discussion, it is evident that much work remains to be done in order to determine if subtle metabolic differences between lean and obese people can help account for the fact that some persons can remain lean in an environment that seems to have been designed to produce obesity.

REFERENCES

1. Abraham, S., and Johnson, C. L. (1980): Prevalance of severe obesity in adults in the United States. *Am. J. Clin. Nutr.*, 33:364–369.
2. Anand, B. K., and Brobeck, J. R. (1951): Hypothalamic control of food intake in rats and cats. *Yale J. Biol. Med.*, 24:123–140.
3. Brobeck, J. R., Tepperman, J., and Long, C. N. H. (1943): Experimental hypothalamic hyperphagia in the albino rat. *Yale J. Biol. Med.*, 15:831–853.
4. Burman, K. D., Latham, K. R., Djuh, Y. Y., Smallbridge, R. C., Yueh-Chu, L. T., Lukes, Y. G., Maunder, R., and Wartofsky, L. (1980): Solubilized nuclear thyroid hormone receptors in circulating human mononuclear cells. *J. Clin. Endocrinol. Metab.*, 51:106–116.
5. Contaldo, F., Presta, E., di Biase, G., Scalfi, L., Mancini, M., Maddalena, G., de Divitiis, O., and Rocco, P. (1981): Preliminary evidence for brown fat defect in human obesity. In: *The Body Weight Regulatory System: Normal and Disturbed Mechanisms*, edited by L. A. Cioffi, W. P. T. James, and T. B. Van Itallie, pp. 143–146. Raven Press, New York.
6. Danforth, E., Jr., Horton, E. S., and Sims, E. A. H. (1981): Nutritionally-induced alterations in thyroid hormone metabolism. In: *13th Miles International Symposium: Nutritional Factors: Modulating Effects on Metabolic Processes*, edited by R. F. Beers, Jr., and E. G. Bassett, pp. 139–153. Raven Press, New York.
7. Deutsch, J. A., Gonzalez, M. F., and Young, W. G. (1980): Two factors control meal size. *Brain Res. Bull.*, 5:Suppl.4, 55–57.
8. Deutsch, J. A. (1978): The stomach in food satiation and the regulation of appetite. *Prog. Neurobiol.*, 10:135–153.
9. Di Rocco, R. J., Yoemans, J. S., and Van Itallie, T. B. (1980): Insulin does not enhance uptake of ^{14}C-deoxyglucose in the ventromedial nucleus of the hypothalamus. *Brain Res. Bull.*, 5:Suppl. 4, 43–54.
10. Ellis, F. R., and Montegriffo, V. M. E. (1970): Veganism: Clinical findings and investigations. *Am. J. Clin. Nutr.*, 23:249–255.
11. Falck, B., and Hillarp, N. A. (1959): On the cellular localization of catecholamines in the brain. *Acta Anat. (Basel)*, 38:277–279.
12. Foster, D. O., and Frydman, M. L. (1978): Nonshivering thermogenesis in the rat: II. Measurements of blood flow with microspheres point to brown adipose tissue as the dominant site of the calorigenesis induced by noradrenaline. *Can. J. Physiol. Pharmacol.*, 56:110–122.

13. Gale, S. K., Van Itallie, T. B., and Faust, I. M. (1981): Effects of palatable diets on body weight and adipose tissue cellularity in the adult obese female Zucker rat (fa/fa). *Metabolism*, 30:105–110.
14. Garattini, S. (1977): Importance of serotonin for explaining the action of some anorectic agents. In: *Recent Advances in Obesity Research: II*, edited by G. Bray, pp. 433–441. Newman Publishing, London.
15. Garrow, J. S. (1981): Thermogenesis and obesity in man. In: *Recent Advances in Obesity Research: III*, edited by P. Björntorp, M. Cairella, and A. N. Howard, pp. 208–213. John Libbey, London.
16. Gurr, M. I., Mawson, R., Rothwell, N. J., and Stock, M. J. (1980): Effects of manipulating dietary protein and energy intake on energy balance and thermogenesis in the pig. *J. Nutr.*, 110:532–542.
17. Hashim, S. A., and Van Itallie, T. B. (1965): Studies in normal and obese subjects with a monitored food dispensing device. *Ann. NY Acad. Sci.*, 131:654–661.
18. Hetherington, A. W., and Ranson, S. W. (1939): Experimental hypothalamico-hypophyseal obesity in the rat. *Proc. Soc. Exp. Biol. Med.*, 41:465–466.
19. Himms-Hagen, J. (1981): Nonshivering thermogenesis, brown adipose tissue, and obesity. In: *13th Miles International Symposium: Nutritional Factors: Modulating Effects on Metabolic Processes*, edited by R. F. Beers, Jr., and E. G. Bassett, pp. 85–99. Raven Press, New York.
20. Hoebel, B. G. (1971): Feeding. Neural control of intake. *Annu. Rev. Physiol.*, 33:533–568.
21. James, W. P. T., and Trayhurn, P. (1981): Obesity in mice and men. In: *13th Miles International Symposium: Nutritional Factors: Modulating Effects on Metabolic Processes*, edited by R. F. Beers, Jr., and E. G. Bassett, pp. 123–138. Raven Press, New York.
22. James, W. P. T., Trayhurn, P., and Garlick, P. (1981): The metabolic basis of subnormal thermogenesis in obesity. In: *Recent Advances in Obesity Research, III*, edited by P. Björntorp, M. Cairella, and A. N. Howard, pp. 220–227. John Libbey, London.
23. Kissileff, H. R., Pi-Sunyer, F. X., Thornton, J., and Smith, G. P. (1981): C-terminal octapeptide of cholecystokinin decreases food intake in man. *Am. J. Clin. Nutr.*, 34:154–160.
24. Landsberg, L., and Young, J. B. (1981): Diet-induced changes in sympathetic nervous system activity. In: *13th Miles International Symposium: Nutritional Factors: Modulating Effects on Metabolic Processes*, edited by R. F. Beers, Jr., and E. G. Bassett, pp. 155–174. Raven Press, New York.
25. Liebling, D. S., Eisner, J. D., Gibbs, J., and Smith, G. P. (1975): Intestinal satiety in rats. *J. Comp. Physiol. Psychol.*, 89:955–965.
26. Lundberg, D., Nelson, R., Wahner, H., and Jones, J. (1976): Protein metabolism in the black bear before and during hibernation. *Mayo Clin. Proc.*, 51:716–722.
27. McCracken, K. J., and Gray, R. (1976): A futile energy cycle in adult rats given a low protein diet at high levels of energy intake. *Proc. Nutr. Soc.*, 35:59A–60A.
28. McHugh, P. R., Moran, T. H., and Barton, G. N. (1975): Satiety: A graded behavioral phenomenon regulating caloric intake. *Science*, 190:167–169.
29. McHugh, P. R. (1979): Aspects of the control of feeding: application of quantitation in psychobiology. *Johns Hopkins Med. J.*, 144:147–155.
30. Miller, D. S., and Payne, P. R. (1962): Weight maintenance and food intake. *J. Nutr.*, 78:255–262.
31. Mogenson, G. J. (1974): Changing views of the role of the hypothalamus in the control of ingestive behaviors. In: *Recent Studies of Hypothalamic Function*, edited by K. Lederis and K. E. Cooper, pp. 268–293. Karger, Basel.
32. Mrosovsky, N. (1981): Body fat during pregnancy and lactation. In: *The Body Weight Regulation System: Normal and Disturbed Mechanisms*, edited by L. A. Cioffi, W. P. T. James, and T. B. Van Itallie, pp. 253–257. Raven Press, New York.
33. Neuman, R. O. (1902): Experimentelle Beitrage zur Lehre von dem Täglichen Nahrungsbedarf des Menschen unter besonderer Berücksichtigung der notwendigan Eiweissmenge. *Arch. Hygiene*, 45:1–87.
34. Nicholls, D. G. (1979): Brown adipose tissue mitochondria. *Biochim. Biophys. Acta*, 549:1–29.
35. Nishizawa, T., Akaoka, I., Nashida, Y., Kawaguchi, Y., Hayashi, E., and Yoshimura, T. (1976): Some factors related to obesity in the Japanese sumo wrestler. *Am. J. Clin. Nutr.*, 29:1167–1174.
36. Paintal, A. S. (1954): A study of gastric stretch receptors: Their role in the peripheral mechanism of satiation of hunger and thirst. *J. Physiol. (Lond.)*, 126:255.
37. Perkins, M. N., Rothwell, N. J., Stock, M. J., and Stone, T. W. (1981): Activation of brown adipose tissue thermogenesis by electrical stimulation of the ventromedial hypothalamus. *J. Physiol. (Lond.)*, 310:32P–33P.

38. Pollock, M. L., Gettman, L. R., Jackson, A., Ayres, J., Ward, A., and Linnerud, A. C. (1977): Body composition of elite class distance runners. *Ann. NY Acad. Sci.*, 301:361–370.

39. Porikos, K. P. (1981): Control of food intake in man: Response to covert caloric dilution of a conventional and palatable diet. In: *The Body Weight Regulatory System: Normal and Disturbed Mechanisms*, edited by L. A. Cioffi, W. P. T. James, and T. B. Van Itallie, pp. 83–87. Raven Press, New York.

40. Porikos, K. P., Hesser, M., and Van Itallie, T. B. (1982): Caloric regulation in nonobese men maintained on a palatable diet of conventional foods. *Physiol. Behav., (in press)*.

41. Rolls, B. J., Rolls, E. T., and Row, E. A. (1979): Sensory specific satiety and appetite. *Int. J. Obes.*, 3:397–398.

42. Rolls, E. T. (1975): *The Brain and Reward*. Pergamon Press, Oxford.

43. Rolls, E. T. (1976): Neurophysiology of feeding. In: *Appetite and Food Intake*, edited by T. Silverstone, pp. 2–42. Dahlem Konferenzen, Berlin.

44. Rothwell, N. J., and Stock, M. J. (1980): Intra-strain differences in the response to overfeeding in the rat. *Proc. Nutr. Soc.*, 39:20A.

45. Rothwell, N. J., and Stock, M. J. (1981): Hyperphagia, thermogenesis and leanness. In: *Recent Advances in Obesity Research: III*, edited by P. Björntorp, M. Cairella, and A. N. Howard, pp. 214–219. John Libbey, London.

46. Rothwell, N. J., and Stock, M. J. (1981): Thermogenesis: Comparative and evolutionary considerations. In: *The Body Weight Regulatory System: Normal and Disturbed Mechanisms*, edited by L. A. Cioffi, W. P. T. James, and T. B. Van Itallie, pp. 335–343. Raven Press, New York.

47. Sanders, T. A. B., Ellis, F. R., and Dickerson, J. W. T. (1978): Studies of vegans: The fatty acid composition of plasma choline phosphyglycerides, erythrocytes, adipose tissue, and breast milk, and some indicators of susceptibility to ischemic heart disease in vegans and omnivore controls. *Am. J. Clin. Nutr.*, 31:805–813.

48. Sclafani, A., and Springer, D. (1976): Dietary obesity in adult rats: Similarities to hypothalamic and human obesity syndromes. *Physiol. Behav.*, 17:461–471.

49. Sclafani, A., and Berner, C. N. (1977): Hyperphagia and obesity produced by parasagittal and coronal hypothalamic knife cuts: Further evidence for a longitudinal feeding inhibitory pathway. *J. Comp. Physiol. Psychol.*, 91:1000–1018.

50. Sherry, D. (1981): Adaptive changes in body weight. In: *The Body Weight Regulatory System: Normal and Disturbed Mechanisms*, edited by L. A. Cioffi, W. P. T. James, and T. B. Van Itallie, pp. 161–168. Raven Press, New York.

51. Smith, G. P., and Gibbs, J. (1976): Cholecystokinin and satiety: Theoretic and therapeutic implications. In: *Hunger: Basic Mechanisms and Clinical Implications*, edited by D. Novin, W. Wyrwicka, and G. Bray, pp. 349–353. Raven Press, New York.

52. Smith, G. P., and Gibbs, J. (1979): Postprandial satiety. In: *Progress in Physiological Psychology and Psychobiology*, edited by J. D. Sprague and A. N. Epstein, pp. 179–242. Academic Press, New York.

53. Stellar, E. (1976): The CNS and appetite: Historical introduction. In: *Appetite and Food Intake*, edited by T. Silverstone, pp. 15–20. Dahlem Konferenzen, Berlin.

54. Stock, M. J., and Rothwell, N. J. (1981): Diet-induced thermogenesis: A role for brown adipose tissue. In: *13th Miles International Symposium: Nutritional Factors: Modulating Effects on Metabolic Processes*, edited by R. F. Beers, Jr., and E. G. Bassett, pp. 101–113. Raven Press, New York.

55. Thurlby, P. L., and Trayhurn, P. (1980): Regional blood flow in genetically obese (ob/ob) mice. The importance of brown adipose tissue to the reduced energy expenditure of non-shivering thermogenesis. *Pfluegers Arch.*, 385:193–202.

55a. Trayhurn, P., and James, W. P. T. (1981): Thermogenesis: Dietary and non-shivering aspects. In: *The Body Weight Regulatory System: Normal and Disturbed Mechanisms*, edited by L. A. Cioffi et al., Raven Press, New York.

56. Van Itallie, T. B., Beaudoin, R., and Mayer, J. (1953): Arteriovenous glucose differences, metabolic hypoglycemia and food intake in man. *J. Clin. Nutr.*, 1:208.

57. Van Itallie, T. B., Gale, S. K., and Kissileff, H. R. (1978): Control of food intake in the regulation of depot fat, an overview. In: *Advances in Modern Nutrition, Vol. 2: Diabetes, Obesity and Vascular Disease: Metabolic and Molecular Interrelationships*, edited by H.M. Katzen and R. J. Mahler, pp. 427–492. Hemisphere Publishing Corporation, John Wiley and Sons, New York.

58. Van Itallie, T. B., and VanderWeele, D. A. (1981): The phenomenon of satiety. In: *Recent Advances in Obesity Research: III*, edited by P. Björntorp, M. Cairella, and A. N. Howard, pp. 278–289. John Libbey, London.
59. Woo, R., Kissileff, H. R., and Pi-Sunyer, F. X. (1979): Is insulin a satiety hormone? *Fed. Proc.*, 38:547.

Health and Obesity, edited by H. L. Conn, Jr.,
E. A. DeFelice, and P. Kuo. Raven Press,
New York © 1983.

Metabolic Abnormalities of Overweight Atherosclerotic Patients

Peter T. Kuo

Department of Medicine, Division of Cardiovascular Diseases, University of Medicine and Dentistry of New Jersey, Rutgers Medical School, Piscataway, New Jersey 08854

Obesity or overweight is one of the most common metabolic disorders of developed nations (8). If obesity is defined as body mass of 20% or greater than average ideal weight for one's height, age, and sex, then it is estimated that between 25 to 45% of the American adult population (14) is overweight. Other methods used to assess the overweight problem include the determination of (a) number and size of fat cells and (b) metabolic disorders associated with obesity. The proposed criteria to define obesity with allowance for some overlapping features between them are listed in Table 1.

An association between obesity and cardiopulmonary disease has been suggested for a long time (3,10,29), but there is much controversy on whether obesity per se is directly responsible for the development of cardiopulmonary diseases. It appears that obesity has to attain massive or morbid proportions (average overweight of 45% or greater than the ideal level) before it can exert a significant deleterious effect on circulatory hemodynamics and pulmonary ventilation, and to contribute directly to cardiopulmonary decompensation and mortality. However, the number of such grossly overweight patients with cardiovascular disease and pulmonary insufficiency is relatively low.

This chapter will direct attention to metabolic disorders in patients with moderate weight gain after adulthood. It is believed that in the attempt to control metabolic abnormalities in prevention of cardiovascular complications of this subset of obesity, emphasis may have to be placed on the early diagnosis of adult-onset and mildly overweight subjects manifesting a group of metabolic disturbances including hyperinsulinemia, glucose intolerance, elevation of low density lipoproteins, and depression of high density lipoproteins. Many of these patients also have mild to

TABLE 1. *Proposed criteria to define obesity[a]*

1) Body mass >20% average ideal weight
2) Fat cell hypertrophy, hyperplasia, or both
3) Metabolic disorders of obesity

[a]With overlapping of features.

moderate hypertension. This type of overweight patient probably constitutes the great majority of the adult population who show increased susceptibility to atherosclerosis. The characteristic metabolic changes demonstrated in a series of mildly overweight atherosclerotic patients are presented for discussion in the following sections.

PLASMA LIPIDS-LIPOPROTEINS IN THE ADULT-ONSET OVERWEIGHT AND ATHEROSCLEROTIC PRONE SUBJECTS

Plasma lipids (cholesterol and triglycerides) are transported *in vivo* as lipoproteins. It has been shown that certain classes of lipoproteins are closely associated with premature development of human atherosclerosis. In earlier investigations Gofman and Jones reported strong association of triglyceride-rich S_f 12–20 and 20–100 lipoproteins or very low density lipoproteins (VLDL) with atherosclerosis, and good correlation of these VLDL species with obesity (16). Although this interrelationship between hypertriglyceridemia (VLDL elevation), coronary artery disease (CAD), and weight gain was further stressed by Albrink and her associates (1,2), the significance of hypertriglyceridemia in CAD has not been substantiated by epidemiologic studies (17,23). Recent demonstration of an inverse correlation between plasma triglycerides (TG) or VLDL level with the CAD-protective high density lipoproteins (HDL) level (18,31) serves to clarify the role of triglycerides or VLDL in CAD, and to emphasize the importance of interaction between the high (HDL) and lower density lipoproteins (VLDL and LDL) (9,40) rather than the level of a single given lipid fraction or lipoprotein species (12) in atherosclerosis. Indeed, disturbance in lipid-lipoprotein metabolism of overweight subjects is not limited to VLDL and LDL elevations but is frequently associated with low HDL levels (15,38,39).

Since a variety of factors including sex, age, diet, and physical activity can affect lipid metabolism in both obese and nonobese subjects (21), and since obesity can occur in hypertrophic, hyperplastic (5,22), and mixed forms (20), we have utilized a previously reported group of patients who were mildly overweight and had abnormal lipid-carbohydrate metabolism (25) and expanded the group for more detailed studies. This group of patients, 16 males and 4 females between 47 and 62 years of age, was selected on the basis of (a) weight gain in mid to late adult life to approximately 20% above the ideal level of the individual; (b) consistent manifestation of hypertriglyceridemia and moderate hypercholesterolemia while on *ad libitum* diet; and (c) no overt diabetes mellitus or severe hyperlipidemia (serum cholesterol and TG less than 320 mg/100 dl and 1,000 mg/100 dl respectively). Some of the pertinent clinical laboratory features of this series of hyperlipidemic and overweight patients are shown in Table 2. The data show relative uniformity of the patient population with mild to moderate obesity, hypertrophic fat cells, and postheparin plasma lipoprotein lipase activity (PHLPLA) at the low end of normal range. Since the weight gain of these patients was due primarily to fat cell hypertrophy and not to increased fat cell number, their PHLPLA were estimated to lie within the normal range on per cell basis.

TABLE 2. *Clinical and laboratory features of adult-onset overweight patients with coronary disease cells*

Age (years)	Sex (M/F)	B.P. range (systolic/diastolic)	% Ideal body wt. range (mean ± SEM)	Fasting PHLPLA[a] range (mean ± SEM)	Fat cell[b] range (mean ± SEM)
47–62	16/4	140–170/90–105	120.8–125.9 (122.5 ± 2.1)	0.30–0.35 (0.326 ± 0.011)	0.669 ± 0.745 (0.699 ± 0.029)

[a]PHLPLA indicates postheparin plasma lipoprotein lipase activity expressed in micro equivalent of free fatty acid (FFA) release per dl per min.
[b]Fat cell expressed as micrograms of lipid per cell.

Their blood pressure was mild to moderately high. Their plasma lipid patterns were quite similar to each other. All of them showed moderately increased serum cholesterol and TG and depressed HDL-cholesterol (HDL-C) levels. These data are presented in Table 3.

RESPONSES TO ORAL GLUCOSE TEST

In preparing patients for oral glucose test, each patient was given detailed instructions to eat a standardized mixed diet with carbohydrate content estimated to provide approximately 50 to 60% of total daily calories for 2 or more weeks until the patient's metabolism and serum lipid levels had stabilized.

Blood Glucose and Plasma Free Fatty Acid

None of the patients had hyperglycemia in the fasting state. Their mean blood glucose levels following ingestion of standard test meals were significantly higher than those of nonobese normolipemic controls for 2 hr. The mean blood glucose level of these patients was lower than their fasting value by the 3rd hr (Table 4).

The mean fasting free fatty acid (FFA) of these 20 patients was only slightly higher, but not significantly higher, than that of controls. The mean ± SEM values of patients were 0.62 ± 0.03 meq/L versus 0.58 ± 0.04 meq/L in the controls. The FAA levels of both the overweight and the control groups were similarly lowered following oral glucose administration.

TABLE 3. *Plasma lipids of 20 adult-onset overweight patients with coronary disease*

Serum cholesterol range (mean ± SEM) (mg/100 dl)	Serum triglycerides range (mean ± SEM) (mg/100 dl)	Serum HDL-cholesterol range (mean ± SEM) (mg/100 dl)
248–305 (299.6 ± 16.2)	298–614 (420.5 ± 54.8)	31–38 (35.1 ± 1.1)

TABLE 4. *Mean ± SEM of blood glucose levels in metabolically overweight CAD patients compared with lean normal controls*

Subject	Oral glucose test (mg/100 mg/dl)				
	Fasting	½ hr	1 hr	2 hr	3 hr
Normal controls (20)[a]	76 ± 3.9	112 ± 4.5	104 ± 6.3	76 ± 4.4	76 ± 3.8
Late-onset overweight patients (20)[a]	70 ± 2.9	139 ± 7.8	147 ± 6.8	108 ± 3.8	67 ± 3.2

[a]Number of subjects in the group.

Serum Lipids and Immunoreactive Insulin Responses

Serum lipids (total cholesterol and TG), basal immunoreactive insulin (IRI), and sums of 3-hr IRI responses to glucose of nonobese normolipemic controls and overweight patients with hypertriglyceride (VLDL elevation) are tabulated in Table 5.

On regular *ad libitum* diets the mean fasting serum levels and that of basal IRI levels of these overweight, hypertriglyceridemic mild to moderate hypercholesterolemic patients were highly elevated above the corresponding level of nonobese normolipemic controls. These overweight patients also exhibited increased IRI responses to glucose stimulation as compared with the control subjects expressed as "sum of 3-hr IRI response" (Table 5).

EFFECT OF HIGH (WITH INCREASED CALORIC INTAKE) AND LOW (WITH REDUCED CALORIC INTAKE) CARBOHYDRATE ON DIURNAL PLASMA TRIGLYCERIDE, FFA, AND IRI ON 10 PATIENTS IN THIS SERIES

Diurnal plasma TG, FFA, and insulin response to diets were investigated in 10 of these overweight hypertriglyceridemic patients. In the first period these patients were maintained on a regular diet with fat, carbohydrate, and protein distributions in 40:45:15% of total daily caloric intake respectively. During the second period, the carbohydrate content was raised by 20 to 25% for 2 weeks while the amounts of fat and protein in the diet were kept unchanged from those of the regular diet used in the initial period of study. In the third 4 to 6 month period, patients were given instructions to keep a low carbohydrate, low calorie diet in which the carbohydrate content was reduced by 15 to 18% of the initial regular diet period level, again keeping the amounts of protein and fat unchanged. The carbohydrate reduction was accomplished mainly by restriction of refined carbohydrates. Monthly follow-up was made on these patients to ensure stabilization of their body weights at reduced levels (20 to 30 lb), before they were readmitted for another round of diurnal metabolic studies.

TABLE 5. *Serum total cholesterol, triglyceride, immuno-reactive insulin (IRI) and IRI responses to glucose test overweight CAD patients vs normal controls*

Subjects	Serum lipids Serum insulin		μU/ml; mean ± SEM	
	Cholesterol mg% ± SEM	Triglyceride mg% ± SEM	Basal	3-hr IRI[b] responses
Late-onset overweight patients (20)[a]	289 ± 16.2	426 ± 55.7	76 ± 5.4	279 ± 37.3
Nonobese normo-lipemic subjects (20)[a]	198 ± 4.6	104 ± 7.0	31 ± 4.8	108 ± 10.1
Between two groups[c]			$p < 0.001$	$p < 0.001$

[a]Number of subjects in the group
[b]Sum of 3-hour serum insulin
[c]Comparison between two groups of subjects.

Blood samples were taken before each meal and at 3-hr intervals over 24-hr at the end of each dietary period for plasma glucose, insulin, FFA total cholesterol (TC) and TG determinations.

Figure 1 shows that, with three regular meals given at 9 a.m., 12 noon, and 6 p.m., the plasma TG curve rises to a plateau spanning the hours between 3 p.m. and 12 midnight then dipping toward the low fasting level at 9 a.m. The whole TG curve is further elevated to reach a peak at 12 midnight after the patients are maintained on a high carbohydrate, high calorie diet for 2 weeks. The abnormally high plasma TG diurnal levels are lowered toward normal with refined carbohydrate restrictive, low calorie diet and weight reduction.

Figure 2 shows "W"-shaped diurnal plasma FFA patterns with patients on the three-meal schedule. All three FFA curves, obtained while the patients were on the three types of diet, are elevated in late afternoon. These curves are suppressed by the 6 p.m. meal and are followed by prolonged elevations lasting throughout the evening fast and extending to the next morning. It is apparent that the diurnal FFA release is increased while the patients are consuming a low carbohydrate, low calorie diet.

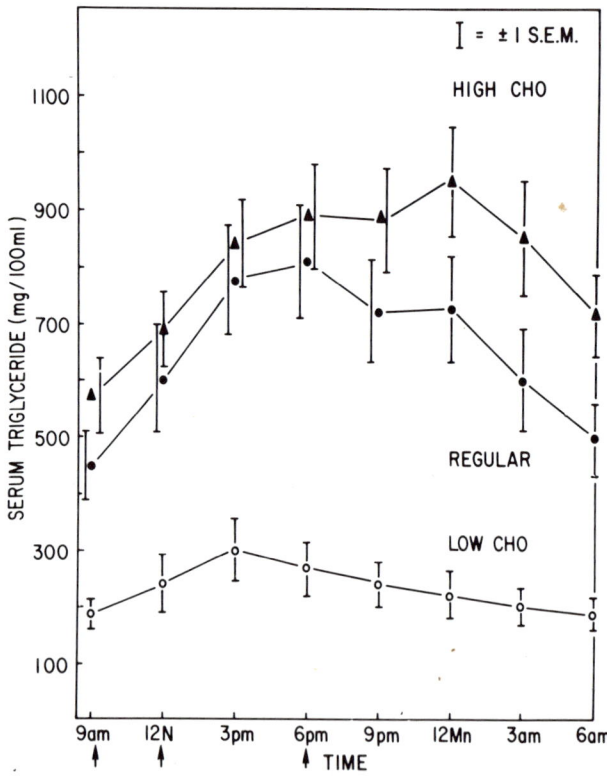

FIG. 1. Diurnal serum triglyceride responses to *ad libitum* (regular) and high and low carbohydrate (CHO) diets. Arrows along the horizontal line indicate the timing of three meals.

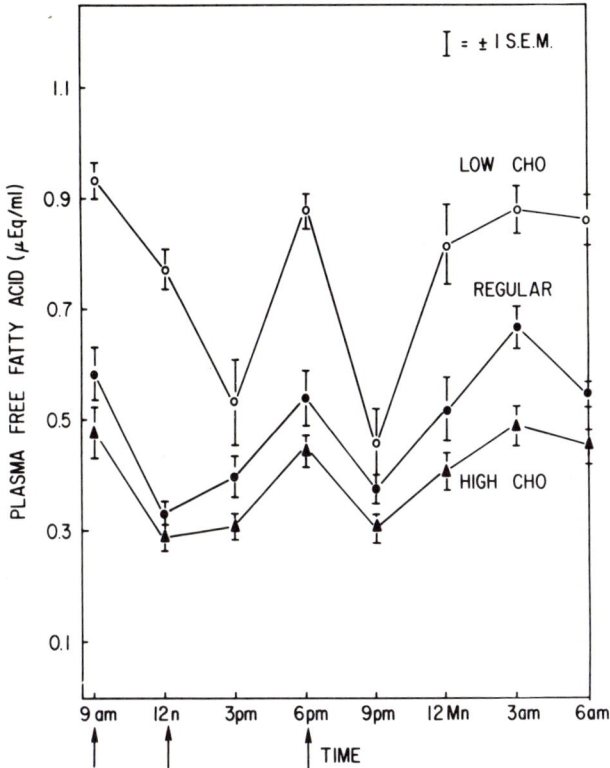

FIG. 2. Diurnal plasma free fatty acid responses to three types of diet and timing of meals as in Fig. 1.

The plasma insulin (IRI) response patterns of these patients to dietary changes show (a) basal hyperinsulinemia while on regular and high carbohydrate, high caloric diets, (b) elevation of serum insulin level with meals, (c) greatly exaggerated responses to high carbohydrate, high caloric diet, and (d) depression of both basal and postprandial levels with low carbohydrate, low caloric intake and weight reduction (Fig. 3).

No dramatic change in the blood glucose values was observed on these 10 patients, while changing from the regular to the low carbohydrate, low calorie diet. As can be expected, their postprandial blood glucose levels were moderately but not dramatically increased with the high carbohydrate, high caloric diet.

TREATMENT OF ADULT-ONSET AND MILDLY OVERWEIGHT PATIENTS

These studies serve to emphasize the need of early diagnosis and control of metabolic abnormalities of a subset of adult-onset and mildly overweight subjects with the hope of preventing the development or to retard and arrest the progression

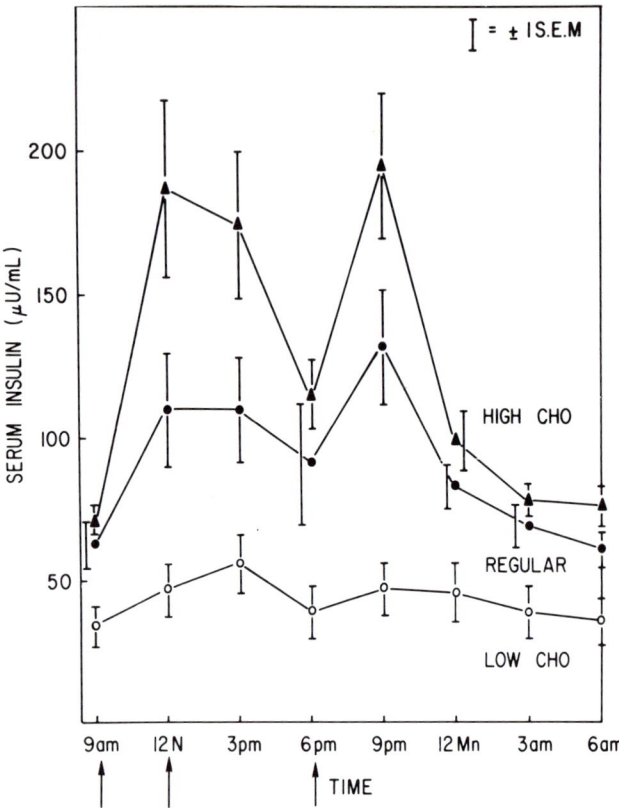

FIG. 3. Diurnal serum insulin responses to the three types of diets and timing of meals as in Fig. 1.

of arterial obstructive disease. Unlike patients with gross or morbid obesity, the metabolic decompensation of this type of obesity can be effectively corrected by relatively minor degrees of dietary restriction. The limited degree of dietary modification helps to boost compliance and to accomplish a lifelong modification of eating habit. It is obvious that successful diet therapy requires the understanding and cooperation of the patient and family, in addition to close follow-up by teamwork of physician, dietician, and nurse. The patient is also urged to follow aerobic exercise regularly (32) at the level to be determined individually by a standardized exercise stress test (30). Physical activity serves to enhance the beneficial effect of diet therapy through improvement of exercise tolerance, as well as in associated metabolic abnormalities and adiposity. The principles of a low simple-carbohydrate, low saturated-fat diet are presented in Table 6.

In general the mild to moderate hypertension of overweight patients improves with diet-exercise treatment. A low dose, long acting diuretic with or without a secondary drug such as a beta blocker or a smooth muscle relaxing agent may be prescribed for the control of persistent hypertension.

TABLE 6. *Principles of dietary plan in the control of metabolic abnormalities of adult-onset mild overweight CAD patients*

Carbohydrate (CHO)
    Constitute about 45% of calorie/day
    Eliminate calorie-dense refined CHO
    Supply carbohydrate calories as starches
       Avoid after meal snacks of dehydrated CHO
Fats
    Constitute ~35% of caloride/day
    Greatly reduced saturated fats and oils
       (Butter, coconut oil, cream, and fatty meat)
    Use unsaturated oils (corn, safflower, soya)
Proteins
    Constitute about 20% of total daily calories
    Generous substitution of fatty meats with fish and fowl
    Use lean cut of meat such as fillet, veal, and shin
Alcohol
    Reduced or restricted (lipemic effect and high calorie)

DISCUSSION

Epidemiological, clinical, genetic, and laboratory investigations have successfully identified a number of risk factors in atherosclerosis. However, with the exception of familial hypercholesterolemia or primary Type II hyperlipoproteinemia (13), the relative importance of each of the risk factors in atherogenesis is still uncertain. In searching for pathogenic mechanism(s) of CAD, a common manifestation of atherosclerosis, up to the present, interest has been mainly directed toward the primary hyperlipidemias (hyperlipoproteinemias). Indeed, the predisposition of patients with several well-defined types of hyperlipoproteinemia to atherosclerosis has been well documented by Fredrickson, Goldstein, and their associates (13). In clinical practice, on the other hand, evidence for a combined disturbance in lipid and carbohydrate metabolism has been demonstrated in a major proportion of atherosclerotic patients (4,35,46). Besides the more subtle hyperlipidemia manifested in mild to moderate hypertriglyceridemia and hypercholesterolemia, these middle-aged patients frequently have decreased glucose tolerance, hyperinsulinemia (41), and increase in fat cell size with truncal adiposity. Practically all of these metabolic abnormalities may be attributable to environmental influence through prolonged ingestion of high carbohydrate, high calorie diets (19,26) in an affluent society and to inconsistent association with positive family history of Type 2 diabetes.

The metabolic studies performed in this series of mildly overweight CAD patients before and after the introduction of dietary perturbations have provided further evidence on the important role of high dietary carbohydrate and calorie intake in inducing a cluster of interrelated metabolic disturbances in adult-onset mildly overweight patients with CAD.

The interrelated participation of the gut, liver, and the adipose tissue in endogenous VLDL (TG) synthesis and release into the circulatory compartment is schematically presented in Fig. 4. Absorbtion of excessive carbohydrate calories greatly

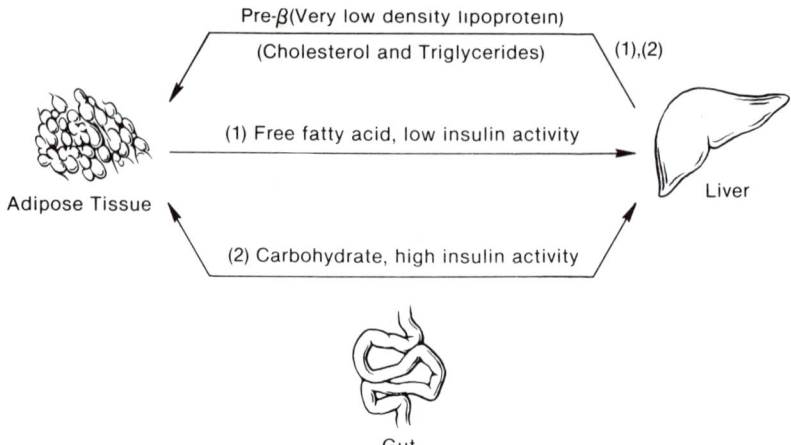

FIG. 4. Schematic representation of interplay between gut, liver, and adipose tissue in VLDL production (hypertriglyceridemia).

enriches the supply of substrates for increased hepatic VLDL (TG) synthesis (34) and release. The limited capacity of the enlarged fat cells to incorporate the TG from TG-rich VLDL would result in its elevation in the blood stream to manifest hypertriglyceridemia in association with moderate hypercholesterolemia. The major pathogenic mechanisms of endogenous hypertriglyceridemia has been demonstrated in this series of overweight patients by a period of high carbohydrate-high caloric diet feeding.

HDL-cholesterol has been negatively correlated with TG concentration, and this has also been related to lipoprotein lipase activity (33). Impaired clearance of chylomicrons and VLDL may decrease the normal transfer of apoproteins and lipids from these LDL species to HDL. In addition, high carbohydrate diet intake would decrease plasma HDL-C concentration and cause a reduction of the HDL_2/HDL_3 ratio (7). On the other hand, plasma HDL-C levels are elevated with increasing degrees of physical activity (27,48).

The key role of hyperinsulinemia in heightened endogenous lipogenesis from carbohydrates is generally recognized. It constitutes one of the major characteristics of this series of adult-onset mildly overweight patient with hypertriglyceridemia (VLDL elevation). The basic hyperinsulinemia and hyperlipidemia are exaggerated with high carbohydrate, high calorie diet; whereas both abnormal metabolic parameters are lowered toward normal with low carbohydrate intake and weight reduction. Although the basic pathogenesis of hyperinsulinemia in obesity is uncertain, investigations made by several groups (19,35,46) are compatible with the contention, that, except for genetic hyperlipidemia, the hyperinsulinemia of the majority of atherosclerotic prone, mildly overweight subjects is environmentally induced through a prolonged period of superimposition of excessive carbohydrate intake on a high caloric diet (24). In line with the induction of hyperinsulinemia by high caloric intake, physical inactivity is known to induce hyperinsulinism, diminished insulin sensitivity, and weight gain (28); whereas physical training lowers plasma insulin and restores insulin sensitivity (6). With regard to the role of hyperinsulinemia in atherosclerosis, a number of clinical studies have reported exaggerated insulin response to oral glucose in patients with CAD or peripheral arterial disease (35,43,46). This association has been substantiated by several prospective studies relating hyperinsulinemia to development of cardiovascular disease (11,37,47). These clinical and epidemiologic studies correlate well with laboratory investigations demonstrating that insulin not only stimulates smooth muscle proliferation in the arterial wall (36,44) but also promotes endogenous VLDL (TG) synthesis (25,42,46).

In reviewing the results of obesity therapy Stunkard and McLaren-Hume (45) reported great limitation in the effectiveness of balanced-deficit dieting in the long-term control of obesity. In our experience the outlook is much brighter in dealing with patients who are not grossly overweight. These patients are usually willing to adopt a relatively easy to follow, moderately restrictive diet, because of awareness of the need to modify their diet on account of symptomatic cardiovascular disease. Long-term follow-up study of a large group of atherosclerotic patients with this more subtle form of obesity may provide information on the efficacy of dietary modification and regulated exercise in controlling the metabolic-hormonal abnormalities and the development and progression of atherosclerosis associated with weight gain after adulthood.

SUMMARY

Pathologic overweight or obesity is difficult to define. We have defined a subset of these patients on the basis of associated disturbances of carbohydrate-lipid metabolism.

These patients are characterized by weight gain after adulthood and development of carbohydrate intolerance, hyperinsulinemia, exaggerated insulin responses to carbohydrates, hypertriglyceridemia or VLDL elevation, depressed HDL level, and mild hypertension.

This subset of mildly adult-onset overweight patients have enlarged fat cells and are susceptible to atherosclerosis.

In these patients, weight reduction, normalization of carbohydrate-lipid metabolism, and hormonal homeostasis can be usually accomplished by restricting the refined-carbohydrate intake and moderating alcohol consumption.

Long-term compliance to the refined-carbohydrate restrictive diet is usually good because it can be tolerated with relative ease, especially by patients with symptomatic cardiovascular disease.

The mild to moderate hypertension associated with weight gain usually improves following the control of the syndromes of obesity. Persistent blood pressure elevation can be controlled by a long acting diuretic with or without a secondary drug such as a β-blocker or smooth muscle relaxing agent.

ACKNOWLEDGMENTS

Supported in part by research grants from Leola Detwiler Teaching and Research Fund and the American Heart Association, New Jersey Affiliate, and Hunterdon-Somerset County Chapter.

REFERENCES

1. Albrink, M. J., Meigs, J. W., Granoff, M. A. (1962): Weight gain and serum triglycerides in normal men. *N. Engl. J. Med.*, 266:484.
2. Albrink, M. J., Meigs, J. W., and Mann, E. B. (1961): Serum lipids hypertension and coronary artery disease. *Am. J. Med.*, 31:4.
3. Berchtold, P., Berger, M., Greiser, E., Dolise, M., Irmscher, K., Gries, F. A., and Zimmerman, H. (1977): Cardiovascular risk factors in gross obesity. *Obesity*, 1:219–229.
4. Bierman, E. L., and Brunzell, J. D. (1978): Interrelationship of atherosclerosis, abnormal lipid metabolism and diabetes. In: *Diabetes, Obesity and Vascular Disease*, edited by H. M. Katzen and R. J. Mahler, pp. 187–210. John Wiley and Sons, New York.
5. Bjorntorp, P., and Sjostrom, L. (1971): Number and size of adipose tissue fat cells in relation to metabolism in human obesity. *Metabolism*, 20:703.
6. Bjorntorp, P., Sjostrand, E., and Sullivan, L. (1970): Effect of physical training on insulin production in obesity. *Metabolism*, 19:631.
7. Blum, C. B., Hall, M., Goebel, R. H., Berman, M., and Levy, R. I. (1976): "See-saw" changes in HDL metabolism with nicotinic acid treatment and carbohydrate feeding. *Clin. Res.*, 24:456A.
8. Bray, G. A. (1976): *The Obese Patient.* In: *Major Problems in Internal Medicine, Volume IX*, pp. 1–43. W. B. Saunders, Co., Philadelphia.
9. Carew, T. E., Koschinsky, T., Hayes, S. B., and Steinberg, D. (1976): A mechanism by which high-density lipoproteins may slow the atherogenic process. *Lancet*, 1:1315.
10. Chiang, B. N., Perlman, L. V., and Epstein, F. H. (1969): Overweight and hypertension: A review. *Circulation*, 39:403.
11. Ducimetiere, P., Eschwege, E., Lapoz, L., Richard, J. L., Claude, J. R., and Rosselin, G. (1980): Relationship of plasma insulin levels to the incidence of myocardial infarction and coronary heart disease mortality in a middle-aged population. *Diabetologia*, 19:205.
12. Førde, O. H., Thelle, D. S., Miller, N. E., and Mjøs, O. D. (1978): The Tromsø Heart Study: Distribution of serum cholesterol between high density and lower density lipoproteins in subjects of Norse, Finnish and Lappish ethnic origin. *Acta Med. Scand.*, 203:21.
13. Fredrickson, D. S., Goldstein, J. L., and Brown, M. S. (1978): The familial hyperlipoprotein-emias. In: *The Metabolic Basis of Inherited Diseases.* edited by J. B. Stanbury, J. B. Wyngaarden, and D. S. Fredrickson, pp. 604–655. 4th ed. New York; McGraw-Hill, New York.
14. *Frequency of Overweight & Underweight*, (1960): Stat. Bull. Metropol. Life Ins. Co., 41:4–7.
15. Glueck, C. J., Taylor, H. L., Jacobs, D., Morrison, J. A., Beagelhole, R., and Williams, O. D. (1980): Plasma high density lipoprotein cholesterol: Association with measurement of body mass. The Lipid Research Clinics Program Prevalence Study. *Circulation*, 62:(Suppl.IV) IV-62–69.
16. Gofman, J. W., and Jones, H. B. (1954): Obesity, fat metabolism and cardiovascular disease. *Circulation*, 5:514.
17. Gordon, T., Castelli, W. P., Hjortland, M. C., Kannel, W. B., and Dawber, T. R. (1977): Diabetes, blood lipids, and the role of obesity in coronary heart disease risk for women: The Framingham Study. *Ann. Intern. Med.*, 87:393.
18. Gordon, T., Castelli, W. P., Hjortland, M. C., Kannel, W. B., and Dawber, R. (1977): High density lipoproteins as a protective factor against coronary heart disease. The Framingham Study. *Am. J. Med.*, 62:707.
19. Grey, N., and Kipnis, N. (1971): *Effect of diet composition on the hyperinsulinemia of obesity.* *N. Engl. J. Med.*, 285:827.
20. Hager, A., Sjostrom, L., Arvidsson, B., Bjorntorp, P., and Smith, U. (1978): Adipose tissue cellularity in obese girls before and after dietary treatments. *Am. J. Clin. Nutr.*, 31:68.
21. Heiss, G., Johnson, N. J., Reiland, S., Davis, C. E., and Tyroler, H. A. (1980): Epidemiology of plasma high density lipoprotein cholesterol levels. *Circulation*, 62:(Suppl. IV)IV-116–136.
22. Hirsch, J., and Batchelor, B. (1976): Adipose tissue cellularity in human obesity. *Clin. Endocrinol. Metab.*, 5:299.

23. Kannel, W. B., Castelli, W. P., and Gordon, T. (1979): Cholesterol in the prediction of atherosclerotic disease: New perspective based on Framingham Study. *Ann. Intern. Med.*, 90:85.
24. Kuo, P. T. (1969): Metabolic basis of human atherosclerosis. *Metabolism*, 18:631.
25. Kuo, P. T., and Feng, L. Y. (1972): Study of serum insulin in atherosclerotic patients with endogenous hypertriglyceridemia. *Metabolism*, 19:372.
26. Laube, H., and Pfeiffer, E. F. (1978): Insulin secretion and the role of nutritional factors. In: *Diabetes, Obesity and Vascular Disease*, edited by H. M. Katzen and R. J. Mahler, pp. 404–409. John Wiley and Sons, New York.
27. Lewis, S., Haskell, W. I., Wood, P. D., Manogian, N., Bailey, J. E., and Perlira, M. (1976): Effects of physical activity on weight reduction in obese middle-aged women. *Am. J. Clin. Nutr.*, 29:152.
28. Lipman, R., Raskin, P., Love, T., Triewasser, J., LeCocq, F. R., and Sojnure, J. J. (1972): Glucose tolerance during decreased physical activity in man. *Diabetes*, 21:101.
29. Mann, G. V. (1974): The influence of obesity on health. *N. Engl. J. Med.*, 291:178.
30. *Manual of Multistage Exercise Test: Protocol for the National Exercise and Heart Project* (1973): *A Cooperative Study*. Social Rehabilitation Service, H.E.W.
31. Miller, G. J., and Miller, N. E. (1975): Plasma-high-density-lipoprotein concentration and development of ischemic heart disease. *Lancet*, 1:16.
32. The National Exercise and Heart Disease Project (1974): *Manual of Operations*. Coordinating Center, The George Washington University Medical Center.
33. Nikkila, E. A., Taskinen, M. R., and Kekki, M. (1978): Relation of plasma high density lipoprotein cholesterol to lipoprotein lipase activity in adipose tissue and skeletal muscle of man. *Atherosclerosis*, 29:497.
34. Olefsky, J. M., Farguhar, J. W., and Reaven, G. M. (1974): Reappraisal of the role of insulin in hypertriglyceridemia. *Am. J. Med.*, 57:551.
35. Peters, N., and Hales, C. N. (1965): Plasma insulin concentration after myocardial infarctions. *Lancet*, 1:1144.
36. Pfeifle, B., and Ditschuneit, H. (1981): Effect of insulin on growth of cultured human arterial smooth muscle cells. *Diabetologia*, 20:155.
37. Pyorala, K. (1979): Relationship of glucose tolerance and plasma insulin to the incidence of coronary heart disease: Results from two population studies in Finland. *Diabetes Care*, 2:131.
38. Rhoads, G. G., Gulbrandsen, C. L., and Kagan, A. (1976): Serum lipoproteins and coronary heart disease in a population study of Hawaii Japanese men. *N. Engl. J. Med.*, 294:293.
39. Rossner, S., and Hallberg, D. (1978): Serum lipoproteins in massive obesity. *Acta Med. Scand.*, 204:103.
40. Schaefer, E. J., Anderson, D. W., Brewer, H. B., Jr., Levy, R. I., Danner, R. N., and Plackwelder, W. C. (1978): Plasma triglyceride regulation of HDL-cholesterol levels. *Lancet*, 2:391.
41. Sims, E. A. H. (1981): Mechanisms of hypertension in the syndromes of obesity. *Int. J. Obes.*, 5, Suppl. 1:9.
42. Stout, R. W. (1977): The effect of insulin and glucose on sterol synthesis in cultured rat arterial smooth muscle cells. *Atherosclerosis*, 27:271.
43. Stout, R. W. (1977): The relationship of abnormal circulatory insulin levels to atherosclerosis. *Atherosclerosis*, 27:1.
44. Stout, R. W., Bierman, E. L., and Ross, R. (1975): Effect of insulin on the proliferation of cultured primate arterial smooth muscle cells. *Clin. Res.*, 36:319.
45. Stunkard, A., and McLaren-Hume, M. (1959): The results of treatment for obesity: A review of the literature and report of a series. *Arch. Intern. Med.*, 103:79.
46. Tzagournis, M., Chiles, R., Ryan, J. M., and Skillman, T. G. (1968): Interrelationships of hyperinsulinism and hypertriglyceridemia in young patients with coronary heart disease. *Circulation*, 38:1156.
47. Welborn, T. A., and Wearne, K. (1972): Coronary heart disease incidence and cardiovascular mortality in Basselton with reference to glucose and insulin concentrations. *Diabetes Care*, 2:154.
48. Wood, P. D., Klein, H., Lewis, S., and Haskell, W. L. (1976): The distribution of plasma lipoproteins in middle-aged male runners. *Metabolism*, 25:1249.

Health and Obesity, edited by H. L. Conn, Jr.,
E. A. DeFelice, and P. Kuo. Raven Press,
New York © 1983.

Diet and Exercise as Treatment for Obesity

George A. Bray

*Department of Medicine, University of Southern California School of Medicine,
Los Angeles, California 90033*

Obesity is a common problem in all affluent societies. Estimates of the number of overweight individuals in the United States vary from 10 to 50 million, depending on the criteria used (9). Using 20% above desirable weight as an index of obesity, the recent prevalence data for this country show that 24% of the women and 14% of men aged 18 to 74 are overweight (12). These numbers indicate that at least 16.3 million American women and 8.5 million American men are significantly overweight. The importance of these data lies in the associated medical and social risks and the current social setting which says that "thin is in."

In the recently promulgated Dietary Guidelines for Americans, individuals are adivsed to "maintain ideal weights" (32). The difficulty comes in putting this sound dietary advice into practice. Anyone who has tried knows how difficult it can be to translate this recommendation into action. Since treatment is so often difficult, prevention would be preferable, and in no field is the old adage that "an ounce of prevention is worth a pound of cure" more apt than in obesity. As yet, however, we don't know how to prevent obesity, nor can we accurately identify obese individuals before they become obese. The best we can do is to identify families where both parents are fat, but even then not more than 80% of the children will be obese (11). For this reason much effort is directed toward treatment. In this chapter I will focus on diet and exercise as treatment for obesity.

ENERGY BALANCE: THE RATIONALE FOR DIET AND EXERCISE

Energy Intake

An increase in body fat reflects an increase in total stored energy measured as joules or calories. Thus excess fat occurs because there is an imbalance between energy (joules or calories) ingested in food and the energy utilized for daily needs (28). For many people body weight remains within a few kilograms over many years suggesting that the body regulates its storage of energy. Given free access to food, this implies that some components of total stored energy or of body size may be controlled.

Food intake occurs during meals, which are separated by intermeal periods when no eating occurs. These meal times are largely determined by environmental factors but the type and quantity of food eaten at a meal have both environmental and physiological controls. Several regions of the brain can influence patterns of food intake. Interest in the hypothalamus arose from the observation that bilateral destruction of the ventromedial hypothalamus in animals and man produced a constellation of changes that included hyperphagia (20). The increased food intake is followed by a rise in body weight and obesity. The way in which the ventromedial hypothalamus modulates caloric balance, however, is unknown.

Short-term regulation of eating appears to be integrated in the lateral hypothalamus. Destructive lesions in this region of the brain decrease food intake and total aphagia may result (16). Conversely, electrical stimulation of the lateral hypothalamus increases food intake. Inhibition of food intake by the hungry animals occurs when isoproterenol, a beta-adrenergic drug, is injected into the lateral hypothalamus. On the other hand, application of norepinephrine to the ventromedial hypothalamus will stimulate food intake in the satiated rat, an effect which is blocked by phentolamine, an alpha-adrenergic blocking drug. These data indicate that adrenergic receptors in the medial and lateral hypothalamus may play a role in the modulation of food-seeking activity.

In addition to the mechanisms in the central nervous system, there appear to be peripheral signals that regulate the onset, duration, and termination of food ingestion (14). Initiation of the next meal may be related, in part, to the size of the stomach. If the stomach is distended, initiation of the next meal may be delayed. Conversely, if the stomach is empty the interval between meals may be shortened. Animals also regulate the quantity of food they eat by "detecting" its energy content. If nondigestible material is added to food, rats will increase the bulk of ingested food in order to maintain a constant total energy intake. Only with very severe dilution of food does this system decompensate (1).

Both neural and humoral factors probably participate in the termination of meals. Since energy stored in triacylglycerol is derived from dietary fat, carbohydrate, and protein, it is likely that circulating levels of amino acids, glucose, fatty acids, and glycerol play a role in signaling the quantity of stored energy. Glucose has received the most attention because it is carefully regulated. Oral or intraperitoneal administration of glucose reduces food intake. On the other hand, blockade of glucose utilization with 2-deoxyglucose enhances food intake. In all likelihood, however, glucose utilization represents only one component of the metabolic process that is recognized by the body as an index of stored energy. Glycerol injected peripherally or infused into the cerebral ventricle reduces food intake (21). No effect of oral glycerol has been found on food intake in human studies (34).

Hormones may also serve in the short-term control of food intake. Injections of insulin will increase hunger and food intake and, if continued, obesity will develop. A possible mechanism for the long-term regulation of body weight involving insulin has been proposed, suggesting that the hypothalamus may respond to the ratio of insulin to growth hormone. The higher the ratio, the greater the quantity of body fat. Insulin may also have an effect through its concentration in the cerebrospinal fluid (45). Glucagon also has an effect but it is opposite to that of insulin—that is, glucagon reduces food intake. Finally, injections of cholecystokinin, a gastrointestinal hormone, will suppress food intake in rats and monkeys and possibly in man (42).

In addition to the internal signals that regulate food intake all animals, including man, receive signals or cues about food from its sight, smell, and taste. Indeed, the environmental cues may be more important in controlling food intake in the obese than are internal cues. External factors such as the time of day, the availability of food, the intensity of lighting, and the tastiness of food are among the most prominent cues (46). For instance, obese college males ate more good-tasting ice cream and less bad-tasting ice cream than lean subjects. Data from other workers attempting to verify the importance of environmental factors in obesity have indicated that the interaction of external and internal cues in the control of food intake is complex (44). Nonetheless, the concept that obese people have a heightened sensitivity to external factors in their environment has been applied to the treatment of obesity with a series of techniques known as behavioral modification (53).

More than 90% of the body energy is stored as triacylglycerol in adipose tissue. This tissue has two principle functions: (a) the synthesis and storage of fatty acids (2) and (b) mobilization of fatty acids as a source of fuel (26). The synthesis of fatty acids by adipose tissue is increased in the presence of insulin and is enhanced by eating a high carbohydrate diet or one with an excess number of calories. Small adipocytes are more responsive to insulin than large adipocytes. Circulating triacylglycerols reach their storage site as lipoproteins from which the fatty acids are released by lipoprotein lipase, and then enter the fat cell. The release of free fatty acids from adipocytes is related to the size of the fat cell. Larger fat cells release more glycerol and fatty acids than smaller fat cells, but adipose cells of similar size obtained from lean or formerly obese individuals have similar rates of lipolysis (16).

In the early years of life fat cells increase in both size and number (43). The multiplication of fat cells continues throughout the growing years. After puberty, fat is stored primarily by increasing the size of adipocytes that already exist although the total number may also increase under some circumstances. Thus, when obesity develops in the early years of life, it is almost always "hypercellular" in type (i.e., an increased number of fat cells). Obesity developing in adult life, however, occurs by an increase in size rather than in the number of adipocytes. Adult-onset obesity is thus primarily "hypertrophic" in type, but recent evidence indicates that this distinction is not absolute.

The anatomic difference between hypertrophic and hypercellular obesity is important because fat cells survive a long time (36). Fat cells develop from stem cells of mesenchymal origin and do not contain fat. Once differentiated, a fat cell does not appear to divide to form new fat cells. In experimental animals the half-life of a fat cell is very long. Thus, with changes in body fat, the size of the individual adipocyte varies but there is little or no change in the total number of fat cells. Even marked and prolonged weight loss does not decrease the number of fat cells. Patients with hypercellular obesity thus have a life long increase in the total mass of total cells. In individuals with an increased total number of adipocytes, weight loss occurs by shrinkage of these fat cells but without a change in total number.

Energy Expenditure

Energy expenditure is the other side of the equation that determines whether there is excess energy for storage. In the normal adult, basal metabolism consumes approximately 800 and 900 kcal/M²/24 hr. The rate of basal metabolism is lower in females than in males and declines with age. Approximate levels for various ages and sexes are shown in Table 1 (9). The decline in basal metabolism rate with age is due in part to increasing fat depots. Individuals who maintained a regular program of physical activity during adult life do not have an increase in body fat with age.

Energy expenditure, measured as oxygen uptake, rises following the ingestion of a meal. The thermic effect of food (formerly called "specific dynamic action") may dissipate up to 10% of the ingested calories. It is probably produced by all foods, but protein appears to have the most effect. Recent data suggest that the specific dynamic effect of a single meal may involve brown adipose tissue (30). The "thermic effects" of food are augmented by exercise. An additional 10% of the total calories ingested can be lost by this phenomenon. These thermic effects of food are mechanisms of "inefficiency" in the body. That is, the calories expended through thermic effects are not available for "useful" work. In the obese the thermic effects of food and of exercise are quantitatively similar to those of lean individuals.

EVALUATION OF THE OBESE PATIENT

When an overweight individual seeks medical attention for his or her problem, an evaluation is needed. The first important decision is whether the individual is sufficiently overweight to require or justify treatment. Although it is difficult to assign any medically significant risks to small degrees of deviation from desirable weight levels, it must nevertheless be an appropriate goal for the physician to recommend maintenance of desirable or optimal body weight. Since the risks from

TABLE 1. *Energy requirements in relation to sex and age[a]*

Age	Male		Female	
	(kcal/kg)	(kcal/lb)	(kcal/kg)	(kcal/lb)
11–14	60	27	48	22
15–18	42	19	38	17
19–22	41	18	38	17
23–50	38	17	36	16
51–75	34	15	33	15
>76	29	13	29	13

[a]Calculated from ref. 46.

being 10 to 20% overweight are small, however, the therapies used must also carry minimal risk to the individual.

In evaluating any overweight individual it is appropriate to obtain the following pieces of information:

1. Anthropometric measurements, including (a) height, (b) weight, (c) circumference of the waist, and (d) (if equipment is available) measurements of skinfold, with preference for the subscapular area, followed by additional measurements of the biceps, triceps, and iliac fat fold.

2. Functional status of an overweight individual, including a listing of those complications that are known to be most frequently associated with overweight. (a) Diabetes mellitus should be evaluated from an elevated fasting blood glucose concentration on at least two occasions, the presence of clinical symptoms, or glycosuria. (b) Blood pressure should be taken, preferably in both arms. Values above 140/90 are abnormal. (c) Serum acylglycerol, uric acid, and cholesterol would be reasonable additional measurements. Testing for the presence of gall stones by ultrasonography and the determination of cardiovascular fitness with a treadmill test may also be considered. An algorithm for evaluating the obese patient is presented in Fig. 1 (18). It summarizes the series of measurements that can be made and their interpretation.

After the evaluation is complete, the decision about therapy is next. The appropriate treatment for obesity depends on the risk associated with the degree of excess weight. This can in turn be expressed by using the body mass index (BMI). The BMI is measured as $wt(kg) \div [Ht(m)]^2$ (10). With weight measured in kg and height in meters, the normal values range between 20 and 26. A nomogram for determining the BMI is shown in Fig. 2. A BMI of 30 is equivalent to 30% overweight, a degree of excess weight that is associated with a 25 to 30% extra risk to life. People with a BMI over 40 are at a very high risk and may have up to 11 times the extra risk to life of people with normal weight (24). The risk to health of extra weight goes up along with the rise in body weight. Thus, all treatments to be considered in dealing with obese patients should be evaluated in terms of the degree of obesity and its attendant risk. A table classifying various types of diets is shown below. This decision should rest on the risk of the treatment compared to the relative risk of the obesity. If the BMI is 25 to 30, there is low risk. With a BMI between 30 and 40 there is moderate risk, and with a BMI above 40 there is high risk (Table 1).

There are a number of modalities that can be used for treatment of overweight individuals. Undoubtedly, the safest and most appropriate for those with low-risk patients is the use of diet. We have already pointed out that the accumulation of body fat requires a positive energy balance. This means that more calories have been ingested than are required for basal needs and for physical activity. For this reason, the initial therapy should attempt to redress this imbalance until the appropriate weight level has been achieved. The use of pharmacologic agents as adjuncts to diet in the restoration of energy balance may help reduce caloric intake, but because they are drugs they are higher risk. Finally, under selected conditions,

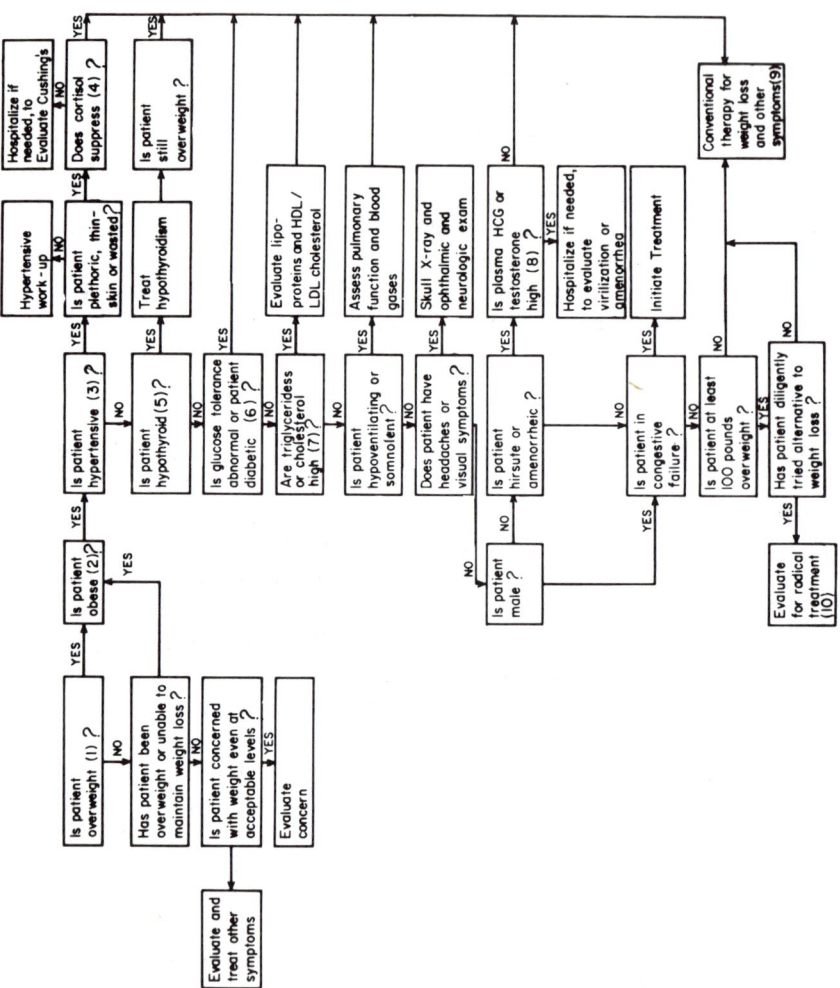

FIG. 1. An algorithm for evaluating the overweight patient. The criteria for abnormality are shown elsewhere (10,18). This reference includes tables for evaluating desirable body weight and body mass index as well as establishing appropriate glucose and blood pressure levels.

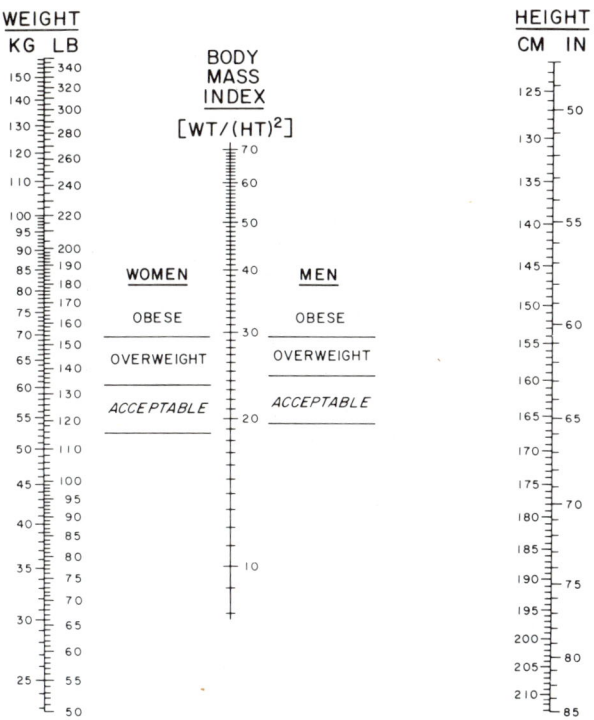

FIG. 2. Nomogram for determining body mass index. A straight edge is attached from the individual's weight on the left side to the point on the right-hand line which corresponds to weight. The body mass index is the point at which this line connecting weight and height crosses the central vertical lines. (Bray, G. A., ref. 10, with permission.)

certain surgical procedures may be considered for high-risk patients. We will deal consecutively with each of these approaches to therapy.

DIETARY TREATMENT

There are four areas to be considered in the use of diet and nutritional education in treating obesity. These are (a) selection of the desired degree of caloric restriction in relation to the person's total caloric needs; (b) the distribution of these calories between carbohydrate, protein, and fat to provide an adequate amount of all nutrients; (c) the frequency with which the foods are to be eaten; and (d) situations in which food is ingested.

Assessment of caloric requirements can be done in one of three ways; the first is to evaluate the patient's age and from Table 1 obtain some estimate of the average caloric need, and then reduce intake below that level. A second and more accurate approach is to use a nomogram (9). With this nomogram it is possible to arrive at a more precise assessment of energy requirements for a particular individual. Use of this figure involves measuring height and weight, determining age, and estimating the relative level of physical activity. The third way to estimate caloric expenditure is from desirable weight tables; for men multiply desirable weight by 33 kcal/kg, for women 30 kcal/kg. Desirable weight can be estimated as follows:

Desirable weight for females = 100 lb + 5 × [height (in inches) − 60]
Desirable weight for males = 106 lb + 6 × [height (in inches) − 60]

After individually assessing daily caloric needs, the next goal is to provide a reasonable caloric deficit. The caloric deficit is the difference between calories required to maintain weight and the calories in the diet. If a calorie deficit of 1,000 calories is maintained, a loss of approximately 7,000 calories will result each week. Since 1-lb of fat tissue contains approximately 3,500 calories, a 1,000-calorie deficit each day will produce a 2-lb loss of fat each week from stores to provide the calories needed for metabolism and activity. In grossly obese people with larger caloric requirements, severe calorie restriction may be unacceptable and realistically unattainable. It is usually best to restrict calories by no more than 500 to 1,000 per day below maintenance levels. Occasionally, however, exceptions to this rule will be necessary.

With adherence to any diet, two phases of weight loss are observed. The first is more rapid than the second and reflects primarily the loss of fluids as the body adjusts to utilizing its stored fat (57). After some days, excess fluid is depleted and subsequent weight loss is slower. After the first 1 to 3 weeks on any diet, many people become distressed with the slowness of weight loss. They may also experience feelings of depression (14). This frustration is compounded by the tendency of some individuals to adapt to caloric restriction by decreasing energy expenditure (5, 28). If this happens, the prescribed diet will produce a smaller weight loss than anticipated, leading to even greater exasperation on the part of the patient. Reassurance and understanding are most important at this time.

New diets frequently appear in popular magazines and in book form (Table 2). This suggests that none of them is ideal; if there were an ideal diet, there would be no need for the continued appearance of new ones. A critique of some of these diets was published recently (4, 25). The low carbohydrate, high protein-high fat diet is a frequently recurring theme. It has been propounded intermittently for more than 100 years. This program raises the question of whether diet imbalanced in one or other of its major nutrients is more beneficial in producing weight loss than a diet that is balanced in all components. Research has provided discordant data on this question. From the results shown in two careful studies, the answer would appear to be "no." In hospitalized patients the fraction of calories provided as fat, carbohydrate, and proteins was varied over a wide range, but, after the initial phase of weight loss due to the excretion of water, changes in the distribution of calories between carbohydrates, fat, and protein had no influence on the rate at which further weight was lost (41, 44). Other studies have suggested that a very low carbohydrate diet may increase the rate at which body fat is catabolized (59). A diet with 30 g of carbohydrate per day was associated with more weight loss than diets with 60 or 104 g of carbohydrate but which were otherwise identical in composition and

TABLE 2. *A classification of diets*

Low calorie diets (above 800 kcal/day)
Balanced diets (contains protein with a proportionate reduction in carbohydrate and fat)
Natural foods (New York Health Department Diet;
Prudent Diet; Weight Watchers Diet; University Diet Plan; Balanced Deficit Diet)
Formula diets (Metrecal; Sego; Slender)
Unbalanced diets
Low carbohydrate (Dr. Atkins Diet Revolution; Dr. Snillman's Quick Weight Loss Diet; The Drinking Man's Diet)
Low fat diets (The Pritikin Diet; The Beverly Hills Diet)
Fad diets that emphasize a single food (The Candy Diet; The Ice Cream Diet)
Very low calorie diets (300 to 800 kcal/day)
Natural foods (The Simeons Diet; The Strang Diet; The Workingman's Diet; University Diet Plan Very Low Calorie Food Diet)
Formula diets
Containing protein carbohydrate and fat (Optifast Program; The Cambridge Diet; The University Diet Formula)
Containing protein only (Liquid Protein-Collagen-Diet; Protein Powders)
Starvation or zero calorie diets

number of calories. The results of this study require confirmation before they can be fully accepted. The long-term consequences to health of a low carbohydrate diet are still open to question, particularly for pregnant women, individuals with kidney disease, and diabetics.

The frequency with which food is ingested may also be important in weight control. The rate of weight loss is not changed by the frequency with which food is eaten (35). However, in normal college-age males, the frequency of feedings did have a significant influence on carbohydrate tolerance and on the level of cholesterol (55). When these men were fed either a weight-maintaining or a weight-reducing diet in one meal, they showed impairment in glucose tolerance and higher levels of plasma cholesterol compared to the same diet fed in three or six feedings. Similar data on cholesterol were reported with obese subjects (8). These data would suggest that it is wise to eat three or more meals per day as plasma cholesterol will be significantly lower and glucose tolerance improved.

How effective are diets in the treatment of obese patients? A summary of the results of dietary treatments for obesity was published by Stunkard and McLaren-Hume (54) and marked a watershed in this field (7). On average only 5% of people who entered diet clinics lost 40 lb and 25% lost 20 lb. There was a considerable difference between clinics in the percentage of people who were successful, i.e., some people are more successful than others in losing weight and the clinical setting seems to influence the results. This implies that behavioral factors that might be termed "motivation" play a central role in the success of any treatment. A more recent review comparing diet with other studies is shown in Fig. 3 (56).

LOW CALORIE DIETS

Low calorie diets are those that provide more than 800 kcal/day (Table 2). These can be divided into two categories: those diets that are balanced and those that

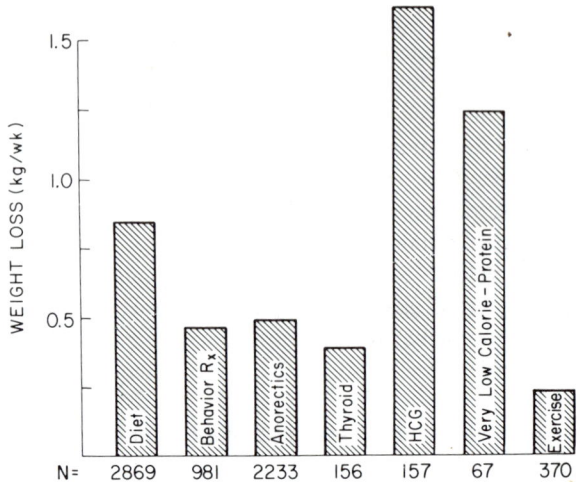

FIG. 3. Rates of weight loss during treatment with various approaches. From refs. 14 and 29a with permission.

TABLE 3. *Median caloric intake by age*

Age (yr)	Male		Female	
	Caucasian	Negro	Caucasian	Negro
1	1,282	1,146	1,162	1,182
2–3	1,504	1,379	1,340	1,360
4–5	1,721	1,647	1,548	1,594
6–7	2,023	1,769	1,784	1,692
8–9	2,097	1,902	1,833	1,645
10–11	2,180	1,877	1,885	1,846
12–14	2,441	2,161	1,858	1,731
15–17	2,890	2,311	1,635	1,601
18–19	2,911	2,482	1,601	1,498
20–24	2,792	2,188	1,580	1,619
25–34	2,591	2,658	1,559	1,352
35–44	2,443	2,144	1,512	1,324
45–54	2,244	1,929	1,465	1,178
55–64	1,988	1,633	1,331	1,156
>65	1,718	1,439	1,254	1,104

From G.A. Bray with permission.

would be generally considered unbalanced (see 37). Balanced diets are those in which calories have been restricted, but where no single food or food substance predominates. The unbalanced diets are those in which one food substance or one type of food predominates. In this latter group are the very low carbohydrate diets (less than 30 g/day) and many other diets identified by special names such as the grapefruit diet, the banana diet, the ice cream diet, the candy diet (Table 3). The unbalanced diet has one major disadvantage and that is the monotony which results when certain classes of food are eliminated. However, these diets may well be unhealthful if continued for a prolonged period. When eating fewer calories than usual, it may be difficult to achieve an adequate intake of all needed nutrients. For this reason I prefer to give all patients supplemental vitamins and inorganic salts.

We have taken two approaches to help our patients determine their level of energy and nutrient intake in their diets. The first approach involves teaching them to "count calories." To do this, we provide the patients with a "monitor" for recording their calories (Fig. 4). These monitors are printed on 3 × 5 cards or pieces of paper that are handy to carry around. Each daily record is kept on a single card so that 7 monitors are needed for each week. On the monitor shown in Fig. 4, they are instructed to write down each food they eat and the amount of that food eaten using weight, volume, or portion size. The calorie value of the liquids and solids are then obtained from a booklet containing calories of foods. At the end of 7 days we have our patients add up liquid and solid calories for each of the 7 days. This information has revealed two important things. The first is the considerable variability from one individual to another in the number of calories eaten in solid or liquid forms. Secondly, for any individual, the variation of caloric intake from day to day has varied by as much as 10-fold. Once individuals have become accustomed to this procedure of "counting calories," some of them like it so well that they use it as a primary technique for controlling and monitoring their weight loss; others, however, find it very difficult to count calories.

Because of the difficulty we have had in getting some patients to carefully and faithfully count calories, we have approached the problem of calorie intake and nutrition by other techniques. The first of these is to use the information that is published on the nutrition label of food packages. A sample of such a nutrition label is shown in Fig. 5. A typical nutrition label shows the serving size and number of servings per container. Below this information are the most important facts for

DAY [ ]	CALIFORNIA DIET PLAN MONITOR FOR CALORIES		
FOOD EATEN	AMOUNT (WEIGHT)	CALORIES SOLID	CALORIES LIQUID

FIG. 4. Form for recording calories. With the use of a calorie guide patients are instructed to record the caloric value for liquid and solid foods that they eat. At the end of the week the totals for each day under the two categories are summarized to give a picture of the entire caloric intake for the week.

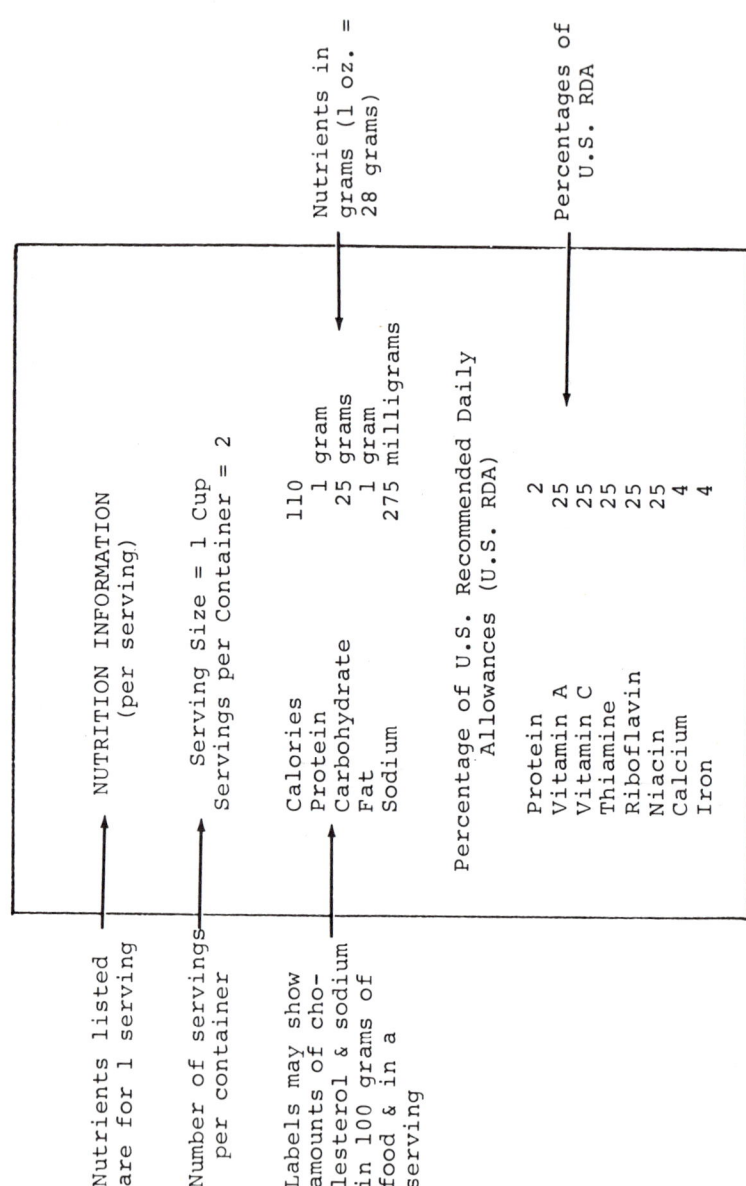

Nutrients listed
are for 1 serving

Number of servings
per container

Labels may show
amounts of cho-
lesterol & sodium
in 100 grams of
food & in a
serving

NUTRITION INFORMATION
(per serving)

Serving Size = 1 Cup
Servings per Container = 2

Calories	110	
Protein	1	gram
Carbohydrate	25	grams
Fat	1	gram
Sodium	275	milligrams

Nutrients in
grams (1 oz. =
28 grams)

Percentage of U.S. Recommended Daily
Allowances (U.S. RDA)

Protein	2
Vitamin A	25
Vitamin C	25
Thiamine	25
Riboflavin	25
Niacin	25
Calcium	4
Iron	4

Percentages of
U.S. RDA

FIG. 5. Nutrition label. This schematic diagram shows the elements that are currently required on labels in which the food is advertised for nutritional purposes. The important information for the overweight individuals is the serving size and the number of calories contained in each serving.

individuals who are counting calories, i.e., the number of calories in a serving in that container. We use the information about protein, carbohydrate, and fat to show that you can calculate the number of calories from proteins, carbohydrates, and fats by using calorie values of 4, 4, and 9, respectively.

With this background information about nutrition labels, we have then tried to deal with calories and nutrients together. Table 4 shows a list of the four food groups on the left, with recommended servings of each per day and examples of a number of foods that can provide these servings along with the major nutrient(s) associated with each group. One of the obvious values of this table is that it shows the wide variation in calories that provide equivalent nutritional servings within each group. For example, skim milk has 90 calories per serving whereas an equivalent nutritional serving of ice cream (1⅓ cups) has 580 calories! The same thing is obvious in the meat group. Peanut butter, for example, provides 400 calories in a serving whereas tuna packed in water has only 75 calories. This table also shows the differences between water- and oil-packed tuna and the variations between different types of meats. After acquainting our patients with these important differences between caloric content and nutrient values of different foods, we provide them with a table that divides food into low and high calorie groups (Table 5). The calorie units we have selected for this purpose are shown below each of the headings. For meats and for fruits and vegetables, we have taken a dividing line of 50 calories per ounce or 50 calories per one-half cup. For the breads and cereals we have taken 75 kcal/serving as the dividing line. For the milk group 100 calories per 8 ounce serving is the dividing line. This table has been a very useful guide for our patients because it can be condensed onto a small 3 × 5 card printed on both sides that can be carried in a pocket as a continuing reminder of the caloric differences and nutrient values.

CHANGING BEHAVIORAL PATTERNS OF EATING

For many of our patients calorie counting, education about food groups, and the use of nutritional contents of foods is not sufficient to help them to lose and maintain their weight loss. For this reason, we have added a variety of behavioral techniques. The basic principles of these behavioral approaches can be summarized under the ABCs of eating. The A stands for *Antecedent*. If one looks at eating as the response to events in the environment, then the antecedent events that trigger eating are of major importance. Eating might be triggered by passing a pizza parlor or entering the home after working or by turning on the television set. Whatever the antecedent may be, it is important for the obese individual and his therapist to come to grips with these antecedents. The B in the ABCs of eating is the *Behavior* of eating. This includes the place, the rate, and the frequency with which an individual eats. It is the actual act of eating. In addition to monitoring the antecedents, we also teach our patients to monitor their eating behavior. Finally, the C in these ABCs is the *Consequence* of the eating, the feelings an individual has about it and, more important, the procedures that an individual can use to provide rewards for changing the pattern of behavior.

TABLE 4. *Table of food groups*

Food group	Recommended servings needed daily	Examples	Serving size	Kilocalories per serving	Major contribution to health
Vegetables and fruits	4	Cooked or canned vegetables, fruits, juices	½ cup	25–100	Vitamins Minerals Fiber
		Raw orange, apple, banana, potato	1 medium	70–95	
		Corn	1 medium ear	70	
		Grapefruit	½ medium	40	
		Cantaloupe	¼ medium	30	
		Raw salad greens	1 cup	20	
Bread and cereal	4	Bread	1 slice	60	B Vitamins Fiber
		Bun (hamburger or hot dog)	½ bun	56	
		English muffin	½ muffin	70	
		Dinner roll	1 roll	60–120	
		Pancake	1 (4 inch)	70	
		Cooked cereals, rice, noodles	½ cup	65–105	
Milk	2 (adult)	Whole milk	8 ounces (1 cup)	160	Calcium
		Low fat (2%) milk	8 ounces	140	
	3 (children)	Skim milk	8 ounces	89	
		Yogurt (plain without fruit)	8 ounces	120–150	Protein
		Cheese	1 ⅓ ounces	120	
		Cottage cheese	1 ½ cups	60	
		Ice cream	1 ⅓ cups	380	
Meat, poultry, fish, and beans	2	Cooked lean meat, poultry, or fish	2 ounces	50–125	Protein
		Hot dogs	2	250	
		Lunch meats	2 ounces (2 sl)	120–190	
		Tuna fish (oil pack)	2 ounces (¼ c)	120	
		(water pack)	2 ounces (¼ c)	75	
		Eggs	2	160	
		Dried beans or peas	1 cup (cooked)	160–250	
		Nuts	½ cup	400–600	
		Peanut butter	4 tablespoons	345	

From G. A. Bray with permission, 1981.

TABLE 5. *Food groups in relation to calories*

Food group	Meat, poultry, fish, and beans (150 kcal/100 g raw)	Milk and cheese (60 kcal/100 g)	Vegetables and fruits (50 kcal/100 g raw)	Bread and cereal
Serving	2	2 (Adult) 3 (Children)	4	4
Relative calorie (energy) value				
Low	Liver Chicken Shellfish: clams, lobster, crab, shrimp, oyster, snapper Abalone Bass Cod Flounder Pike Halibut Swordfish Tuna (water packed) Haddock Perch	Skim milk Low-fat milk Buttermilk Yogurt (skim milk)	Asparagus Beets Brocolli Cabbage Celery Chard-spinach Cucumber Green beans Greens Lettuce Mushrooms Pickles Squash (summer) Tomatoes Turnips Apple juice Cantaloupe Berries Boysenberries Cranberries Lemon Gooseberries Grapefruit Oranges Papayas Peaches Strawberries Watermelon	Bread Melba toast Dry, non-sugared cereals Cooked grain cereals
High	Meats: Beef Ham Lamb Pork Bologna Frankfurters Turkey Veal Egg Fish: Herring Sardines Trout Tuna (oil packed) Salmon Whitefish	Cottage cheese Whole milk Ice cream Evaporated milk Goat milk Cheese	Lima beans Peas Potatoes Sweet potatoes Winter squash Apple Apricots Bananas Cherries Grape juice Grapes Guava Mango Pears Pineapple Plums Prunes Raspberries	Biscuits Muffins Rolls Corn bread and grits Crackers Cookies Pie Pasta (macaroni noodles, etc.) Tortillas Doughnuts

From G. A. Bray with permission, 1981.

The practical approach to eating behavior used in our clinic has been developed over a period of several years based on concepts of Stuart and Davis (53), Jordan et al. (40), and Ferguson (27). We have evolved a stepwise approach to analyzing patterns of eating using 3 × 5 cards similar to the one shown earlier. First, the individual is instructed to identify the foods that he eats and the activities associated with eating or the places where he eats. At the end of each week, the individual determines the cumulative frequency for activities and/or places associated with eating. After completing this analysis, he has some concept of the events and places that are associated with eating. We then make suggestions for changes based on this analysis. For example, if eating occurs primarily when watching television, we point out this association and suggest that he not eat when watching television or change the type of food he eats. We then use the technique of stimulus control to help modify his eating. By stimulus control, we mean reducing the number of places or times and other environmental factors when he eats. This can be done by confining the act of eating to a single place and concentrating on the act of eating itself, rather than watching television. Distracting events of other types are also to be avoided. For many individuals the very act of writing down what they eat and observing themselves eating in this fashion is a unique and valuable experience that by itself initiates changes in eating behavior.

During the next week we have the patient monitor his eating by identifying the meals or snacks. A snack is defined as a single item or two, and a meal consists of three or more items consumed at the same time. Analyzing eating is done by counting the number of meals during each hour and recording it on a graph. The peak times for eating and the rate of eating are thus both presented visually. We encourage patients to consolidate the number of meals or to reduce the rate at which food is eaten. During the ensuing week they make another recording and return to repeat the analysis and observe their progress.

As a third exercise, we have patients record hunger at the time of eating and the taste of the food they eat. The purpose of this exercise is to have each individual spend time judging the flavor of food and deciding whether he was hungry when he began eating. The degree of hunger is rated on a scale of 1 to 5 with 1 equal to not at all and 5 most ever. The taste of food is similarly rated from excellent to poor on a scale of 1 to 5. A number is placed in the appropriate column for each eating event to note the degree of hunger and the taste of the key foods when eating began. After 1 week of recording, the number of times a hunger rating is in each category (1 to 5) is totaled. A similar set of totals are made for taste ratings. The goal is to decrease the amount of eating at times when patients are not hungry and to become more discriminating by eating more foods that they really like. After coming to grips with taste and hunger, we encourage patients to try and eliminate some of those events where they ate without being hungry and to avoid eating those foods that do not taste good. For many of our overweight patients this analysis of the ABCs of eating has been of great value in their ability to control eating. For some these approaches are much more effective than counting calories and for other individuals counting calories is a much more rewarding approach.

EVALUATION OF DIETS

Thyroid hormone has been widely used in the treatment of obesity (9). In 1963 Gordon et al. (31) published a treatment program that received widespread attention. We decided to extend their investigation in order to gain comparative data on the effects of triiodothyronine and placebo treatment. We hospitalized two groups of patients who were fed a 1,320-calorie diet that was started following a 48-hr fast. Doses of triiodothyronine (T3) were increased to a maximum of 125 μg/day and injections of mercurial diuretics were given to both groups. The rate of weight loss expressed as grams per day was calculated after 28 days on this program (Table 5). It is clear that the patients treated with T3 lost significantly more weight. However, there is also valuable information on the effect of placebo treatment, i.e., caloric restriction. These effects will serve as the basis for comparison of other treatments that have been conducted using outpatient subjects over the past 15 years.

The use of T3 for treatment of obesity has also been carried on with outpatients, including a controlled double-blind trial of T3 and placebo published from our laboratory (19). The design was a crossover with two treatment periods of 4 weeks each, with 2 weeks on no medication in between. The T3 (225 μg/day) was given either before or after the placebo. Thus all subjects received both placebo and T3. Weight loss with T3 averaged 140 g/day. During the treatment with placebo there was actually a weight gain of 112 g/day. These subjects weighed an average of 30 to 40 kg more than did those in the study of hospitalized patients. In addition the outpatients were given diets containing 1,000 calories rather than the 1,320 calorie diet used in the hospital. Thus, the smaller weight loss of the outpatient group indicated that they were not adhering to the diet as well as the hospitalized patients and thus use of T3 was not as effective as with the inpatients. Indeed the outpatients treated with T3 lost weight more slowly than the placebo group in the hospital. Moreover the outpatient group treated with placebo actually gained weight whether the placebo came before or after the treatment with T3.

Appetite suppressants are the most widely used group of pharmacologic agents. All of them are derived from phenethylamine except one. Phenylpropranolamine (PPA) is the only member of this group that is available without a prescription. It can be purchased in a variety of different capsules that contain PPA alone or in combination with methylcellulose or caffeine. The oldest of the prescription drugs is dextroamphetamine. In the mid-1930s this compound was incidentally observed to induce weight loss. However, d-amphetamine was associated with significant central excitatory effects and with numerous cases of addiction. The clinically available compounds show considerable variation in the central excitatory effects, but are all appetite suppressants. This dissociation of central excitatory properties has been shown most vividly using EEG tracings in subjects given fenfluramine, amphetamine, and barbiturates. The effects of fenfluramine on the electroencephalogram were like those seen with the barbiturates, and were very different from the effects seen with amphetamines. Thus, the organic chemist has been largely successful in separating the central excitatory properties from the appetite-suppressing activities of these molecules.

Do appetite suppressants work? The evidence supporting the effectiveness of these drugs has been reviewed by Scoville (50) and by Sullivan and Comai (55). In the review of applications submitted to the FDA, Scoville reported that drug-treated patients lost an average 0.51 lb/week (220 g/week) more than the placebo-treated control groups. During the past decade three new appetite suppressing drugs have been marketed. These are fenfluramine (Pondimin®), mazindol (Sanorex®), and clortermine (Voranil®). In two clinical trials we have compared appetite suppressants and placebos against diet and behavioral management. The first trial, which examined a behavioral program without placebo, a placebo, and two appetite-suppressing drugs had two goals. The first was to evaluate predictive factors that might prospectively identify those patients who were going to be successful during the course of the program. Second, we wanted to compare behavioral treatment with drug treatment in terms of weight loss and duration of attendance at the clinic. A total of 120 patients were started on the program and there were no charges for participation. The two appetite suppressants were mazindol and diethylpropion, and each subject received a 1,000 calorie diet. Figure 6 shows the number of patients remaining in the study with time after the initial visits. The dropout rates were essentially identical for the four treatments with approximately one-half of the patients still in treatment after 8 weeks.

Before beginning the specific treatment, each patient completed a variety of pencil and paper tests. The tests included measures of self-esteem, social acceptance, locus of control, responsiveness to external stimuli, attitudes toward weight loss, and knowledge about nutrition. Success was related to social conformity and a desire for social acceptance. Locus of control and self-esteem were not related to success. Individuals who believed that poor eating habits caused their obesity also tended to be more successful. Finally success was more likely in those who were less responsive to environmental cues (48).

Weight loss for the full 14 weeks and for all patients at the time when they dropped out of the program are shown in Fig. 7. Patients in the behavioral program

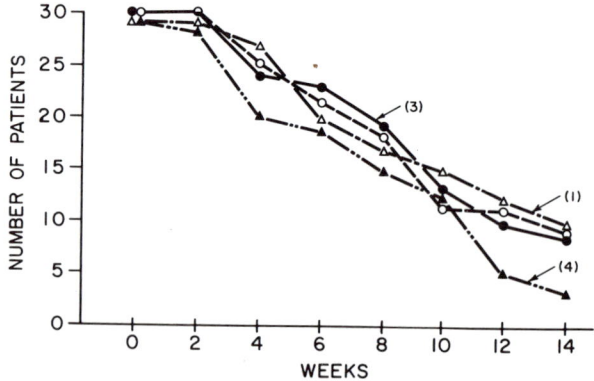

FIG. 6. Drop-out rate from clinic during treatment. The number of patients remaining in treatment each 2 weeks is shown for the mazindol (1), diethylpropion (2), placebo (3), and behavioral change (4) groups. (From Dahms et al., ref. 21, with permission.)

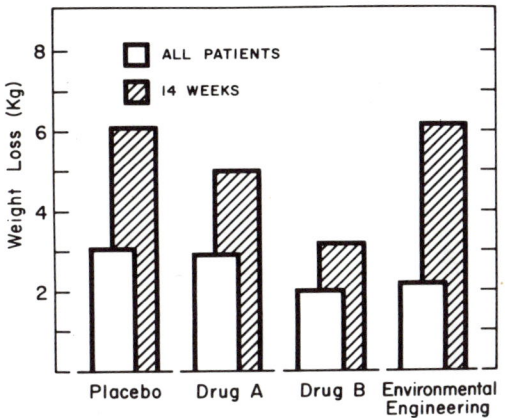

FIG. 7. Weight loss during treatment. The weight loss for those remaining in treatment for the entire time and for the length of follow-up for the remainder is shown. Note that the weight losses by the placebo-treated and behavioral change groups exceeded those of the two drug-treated groups. *Solid bar:* All patients; *hatched bar:* after 14 weeks. From Dahms et al., ref 21, with permission.

and the placebo groups lost weight as well as, or better than, those in the drug-treated groups. These findings strengthened our interest in behavioral change. The success of the placebo-treated groups also intrigued us. On the other hand, the high dropout rate was discouraging because it probably reflected failure for the people who dropped out.

A second study also compared appetite-suppressing drugs with behavioral treatment aimed at changing eating habits. This study had a much more sophisticated design. Each treatment group had 12 patients, 4 on placebo and 8 on drug, and there were 5 replicates of this basic grouping. Each replicate of 12 patients was assigned to 1 of 5 therapists and each therapist thus got a complete block of 12 patients. The use of 5 therapists gave us a chance to address the question of whether physicians or nonphysicians are better therapists. Patients paid a refundable fee for participating in the clinic, whereas the first study had no cost. Patients were asked to pay $50, which was to be returned to them in two installments, one-half at the end of the treatment period and the other one-half 2 months after the end of the study when they returned to be weighed. This study was one part of a broader study conducted in five hospitals. The data from the other four hospitals are shown on the left in Fig. 8 the data from our clinic on the right. All patients in our clinic participated in a behavioral program designed collectively by the 5 therapists. This behavioral component made our study different from the other four clinics, none of which had a behavioral program. In the other clinics, the drug-treated patients lost an average of 6 pounds. Thus, our placebo group lost about four times as much weight as the placebo-treated group in the other clinics. In our clinic the placebo-treated patients lost almost as much weight as the drug-treated patients in the other four clinics. Calculations of weight loss show that drug-treated patients in our clinic lost about 60 g/day and the placebo-treated group 40 g/day (21).

In 1954 Simeons introduced the use of injections of human chorionic gonadotropin (HCG) into the treatment of obesity. Several recent controlled trials of HCG and an appropriate placebo have been conducted to evaluate its effectiveness (33, 52).

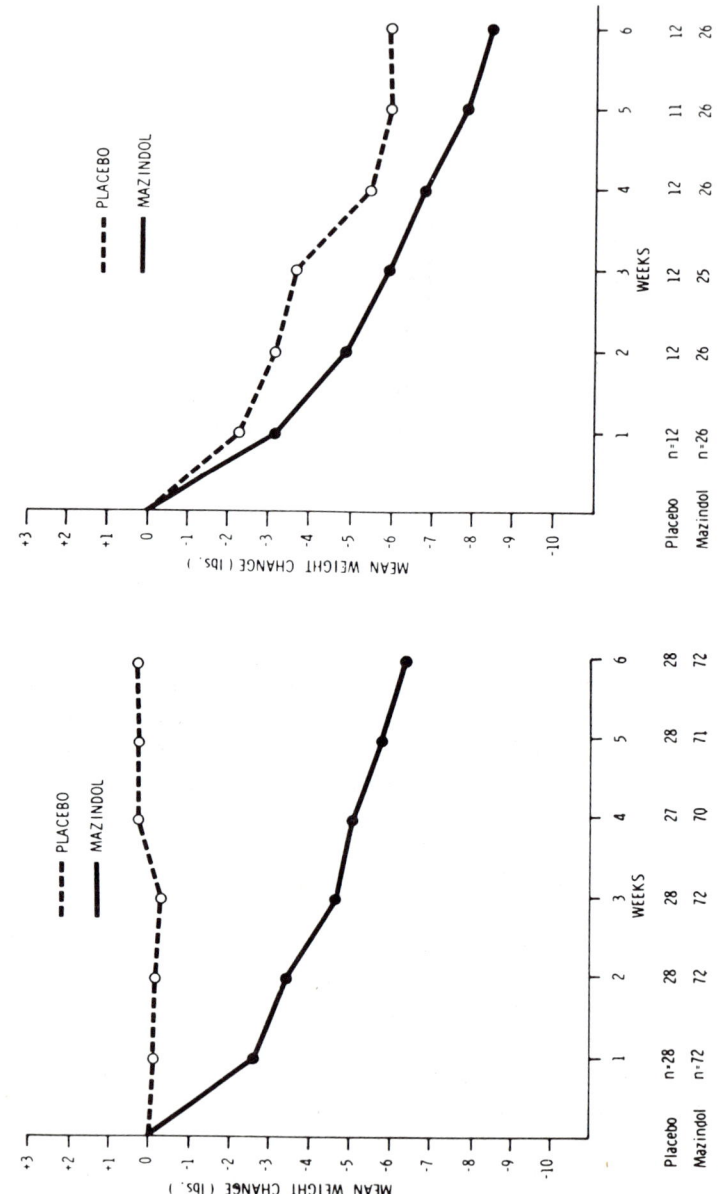

FIG. 8. Weight loss during treatment with mazindol or placebo. The left-hand panel shows the data on the four clinics in which the protocol was used without any behavioral program. The right-hand panel shows the patients in our clinic who were treated with a behavioral program and either placebo or drug. (Adapted from Mazindol data.).

All patients were given a balanced very low calorie diet containing 550 kcal/day. The two groups of patients treated with either placebo or HCG lost weight at almost identical rates; those treated with HCG lost an average of 8.8 kg, and the placebo-treated group 8.1 kg. When calculated in grams per day, the HCG-treated patients lost 210 g/day and the placebo-treated patients lost 193 g/day, both of which are well above the rate of weight loss for any of the placebo-treated patients studied in outpatient trials. These rates of weight loss are close to those of massively obese inpatients eating 1,320 kcal/day. Four other programs using HCG show similarly striking effects (56). Only a few dietary or behavioral studies show such rapid weight loss.

Several general points emerge from this review of modalities used in the treatment for obesity. First, all of the treatments with low risk are successful for some patients. These beneficial effects, however, last for variable periods of time with long-term results that are often disappointing. Like most other chronic problems in clinical medicine, treatment of obese patients is largely a problem in compliance. Some patients drop out in all treatment programs near the beginning but most will achieve some progress toward their goal. Only a small number of patients however will maintain the weight which is lost. Second, the fraction of patients who will achieve weight loss for a long period of time seems to vary from one clinic to another suggesting that such things as the skill and experience of the therapists, the design of the program, and the techniques used to motivate the patient are all important variables. Third, nonphysicians can do as well as physicians under many circumstances. Fourth, the successful patients cannot yet be predicted with any success using pencil and paper tests, but there are some suggestive leads from measurements involving responsiveness to external stimuli.

VERY LOW CALORIE DIETS

The use of very low calorie diets has had periods of popularity throughout this century and are in "vogue" now. Evans and his colleagues more than 40 years ago recommended the use of very low calorie diets as a modality for treating obese individuals. This idea gradually lost favor. However, nearly 20 years later, liquid diets were introduced and became commercially successful. Metrecal® one of the first products had a meteoric rise in popularity and then fell into disfavor. More recently, the use of very low calorie diets in which protein is the principal nutrient have been developed and commercialized in several forms. The evidence is clear that, with all of the programs now in use, patients can lose up to 200 g/day or more. This equals the rates of weight loss seen in patients treated with the chorionic gonadotropin or the corresponding placebo and encouraged to adhere to a 550 kcal/day diet. These very low calorie diets are designed to provide 240 to 700 calories per day (5, 29, 37). Protein comprises between one-third and 100% of the energy. In addition, supplements of electrolytes, including potassium and other inorganic salts as well as vitamins, including folate, pyridoxine, and thiamin are usually given. In the recent past the use of a proteolytic digest of collagen was associated with more than 59 deaths among women, indicating that digested collagen is a high-risk treatment. The Center of Disease Control in the United States has released the data on 16 of these women treated with liquid protein diets who died and for whom no other adequate explanation for death was available. These women ranged in age from 23 to 51 years. Autopsies showed abnormalities of the myocardium with premorbid evidence of cardiac arrhythmias (51). Because of this unfortunate experience with liquid protein diets, it would appear judicious for very low calorie diets to contain not only protein, but some carbohydrate. Diets containing only protein should be avoided since the possibility exists that any form of protein diet without adequate carbohydrate or fat supplements might produce the same untoward reactions observed in individuals fed liquid protein diets.

STARVATION OR FASTING

Undoubtedly, the fastest way to lose body weight is by total starvation but this is a risky procedure (23). In this process, as with any other diet, there are two phases of weight loss. The first phase is rapid and reflects the loss of significant amounts of water as the body adjusts to utilizing its stored fat. After 24 to 48 hr, glycogen stores and the associated water are depleted. Gluconeogenesis from proteins is at a maximum at this time. After the first 1 to 3 weeks of starvation, the rate of weight loss falls below 0.5 kg/day, reflecting the reduced losses of body protein. Several deaths have been reported during therapeutic starvation in obese patients. Equally discouraging have been the long-term results. After weeks to months, most individuals regain weight slowly and in most instances return to their initial weight.

EXERCISE AND PHYSICAL ACTIVITY IN TREATMENT

Another approach to losing weight is to increase energy expenditure. The components of energy expenditure by human beings can be divided into three parts: basal metabolism, heat losses due to thermic effects of food, and the energy needs for physical activity. Basal metabolic needs are slightly lower for women than for men, but in general are approximately 1,000 kcal/M²/day. Heat losses due to thermic effects of food (originally called specific dynamic action) are small and not more than 10% of the caloric value of the ingested foods. The energy needed for physical activity obviously depends on the degree of activity. Since basal metabolism is not subject to significant changes and thermic effects are small, the only part of energy expenditure that is amenable to significant manipulation is physical activity. Table 6 summarizes levels of physical activity and has been adapted from the *Recommended Dietary Allowances* of the National Academy of Sciences (46). The lowest level of activity is slightly less than 0.8 kcal/min. Thus, if an individual sleeps for an entire 24 hr around 1,150 calories will be expended. Reclining increases this level from 0.8 to approximately 1.0 to 1.4 kcal/min. Very light activity (i.e., the level at which people spend most of their waking time) consumes between 1.5 and 2.0 kcal/min. Light activity increases this from 2.0 to 3.5 kcal/min, whereas mod-

TABLE 6. *Weight loss by patients participating in hospital and outpatient studies of treatments for obesity*

Treatment	Dose of drug	Diet (kcal/day)	Duration of treatment (day)	Treated			Placebo		
				Number of patients	Initial body weight (kg)	Weight loss (kg/week)	Number of patients	Initial body weight (kg)	Weight loss (kg/week)
Hospital									
Triiodothyronine	125 µg/day	1,320	28	6	105	1.60	6	109	1.15
Outpatient									
Triiodothyronine	225 µg/day	1,000	28	12	146	0.98	9	146	+0.78
Study 1 Mazindol	1 mg t.i.d.	1,000	84	10	105	0.42		118	0.51
Diethylpropion	25 mg t.i.d.			10	112	0.26	4	114	0.52
Study 2 Mazindol	2 mg/day	1,000	49	24	94	0.63	12	92	0.65
Human chorionic Gonadotropin	125 µ/day	550	42	18	80	1.47	14	80	1.35
Acupuncture	None	None	21	24	66	0.17	—	—	0.0

From G.A. Bray, with permission.

erate activity ranges from 3.5 to 7.0 kcal/min. Only with heavy exertion does energy expenditure rise above 7.5 kcal/min. Few people spend much of their time involved in this level of physical activity. Studies show that the use of exercise alone has produced less weight loss than other modalities (56). It is desirable, however, to encourage patients to increase activity as an alternative to eating (35).

SUMMARY

Although we have examined the elements of treatment in an isolated fashion, it is often possible to provide more than one of these components together. Thus, anorectic drugs can be used along with a well-balanced low calorie diet. Similarly programs focusing on behavioral changes can go hand in hand with education in nutrition and dieting. The use of exercise or other programs to increase movement can be used with any of the programs. From a practical point of view, it seems best to have a multifaceted program in which there are several starting points for different patients. Such a strategy provides the possibility for varying the subsequent treatment program. In our clinic we have four phases that we believe can all be used profitably. We have been impressed with the rapid weight loss and high adherence of placebo-treated groups given small injections of saline in the HCG program. The second and third phases of our program focus respectively on nutrition and behavioral changes in eating. For many patients one or more of the techniques that they learn in such a program can be useful for continuing to lose weight. Finally, we believe that formula diets can be very useful for additional short periods where rapid weight loss is desired. From the work that is in progress in our laboratory there are several possible formulations that provide the essential elements of nutrition as well as help people to lose weight. For some massively overweight individuals this group of low-risk therapies are inadequate. For them the use of surgical procedures is carefully evaluated and when the individual is interested they may be undertaken.

REFERENCES

1. Adolph, E. F. (1979): Look at Physiological Integration. *Am. J. Physiol.*, 237:R255–259.
2. Angel, A., and Bray, G. A. (1979): Synthesis of fatty acids and cholesterol by liver, adipose tissue and intestinal mucosa from obese and control patients. *Eur. J. Clin. Invest.*, 9:355–362.
3. Atkinson, R. L., Greenway, F. L., Bray, G. A., Dahms, W. T., Molitch, M. E., Hamilton, K., and Rodin, J. (1977): Treatment of obesity: Comparison of medical and nonphysician therapists using placebo and anorectic drugs in a double-blind trial. *Int. J. Obes.*, 1:113–120.
4. Berland, T. (1979): Diets '79. Everything you should know about the diets making news. *Consumer Guide Magazine Health Quarterly*, V. 223.
5. Bistrian, B. R., Winterer, J., Blackburn, G. L., Young, V., and Sherman, M. (1977): Effect of protein-sparing diet and brief fast on nitrogen metabolism in mildly obese subjects. *J. Lab. Clin. Med.*, 89:1030–1035.
6. Bray, G. A. (1969): Effect of caloric restriction on energy expenditure in obese patients. *Lancet*, 2:397–398.
7. Bray, G. A. (1970): The myth of diet in the management of obesity. *Am. J. Clin. Nutr.*, 23:1141–1148.
8. Bray, G. A. (1972): Lipogenesis in human adipose tissue: Some effects of nibbling and gorging. *J. Clin. Invest.*, 51:537–548.

9. Bray, G. A. (1976): *Major Problems in Internal Medicine, Vol. 9: The Obese Patient*, W. B. Saunders Company, Philadelphia.
10. Bray, G. A. (1978): Definitions, measurements and classification of the syndromes of obesity. *Int. J. Obes.*, 2:99–112.
11. Bray, G. A. (1979): Obesity. *DM*, 26:1–85.
12. Bray, G. A. (1979): Obesity in America. An overview of the Second Fogarty International Center Conference on Obesity. *Int. J. Obes.*, 3:363–375.
13. Bray, G. A. (1979): *Obesity in America*. D.H.E.W. Publication No. (N.I.H.) 79–359.
14. Bray, G. A. (1981): Nutrition education for physicians in the 80s. In: *Recent Advances in Clinical Nutrition I: Proceedings of the 1st International Symposium on Clinical Nutrition 9–11 July 1980 Royal College of Physicians, London*, edited by A. N. Howard and I. McLean Baird, pp. 263–269. John Libbey and Co., London.
15. Bray, G. A., Dahms, W. T., Atkinson, R. L., Rodin, J., Taylor, I., Schwartz, A., and Frame, C. (1979): Metabolic and behavioral differences between dieting and intestinal bypass. *Horm. Metab. Res.*, 11:648–654.
16. Bray, G. A., Glennon, J. A., Salans, L. B., Horton, E. S., Danforth, E., Jr., and Sims, E. A. H. (1977): Spontaneous and experimental human obesity: Effects of diet and adipose cell size on lipolysis and lipogenesis. *Metabolism*, 26:739–747.
17. Bray, G. A., Inoue, S., and Nishizawa, Y. (1981): Hypothalamic obesity. The autonomic hypothesis and lateral hypothalamus. *Diabetologia*, 20:366–377.
18. Bray, G. A., Jordan, H. A., and Sims, E. A. H. (1976): Evaluation of the obese patient. I. An Algorithm. *JAMA*, 235:1487–1491.
19. Bray, G. A., Melvin, K. E. W., and Chopra, I. J. (1973): Effect of triiodothyronine on some metabolic responses of obese patients. *Am. J. Clin. Nutr.*, 26:715–721.
20. Bray, G. A., and York, D. A. (1979): Hypothalamic and genetic obesity in experimental animals: An autonomic and endocrine hypothesis. *Physiol. Rev.*, 59:719–809.
21. Dahms, W. T., Molitch, M., Bray, G. A., Greenway, F. L., Atkinson, R. L., and Hamilton, K. (1978): Treatment of obesity: Cost-benefit assessment of behavioral therapy, placebo and two anorectic drugs. *Am. J. Clin. Nutr.*, 31:774–778.
22. Davis, J. D., Wirtshafter, D., Asin, K. E., and Brief, D. (1981): Sustained intracerebroventricular infusion of brain fuels reduced body weight and food intake in rats. *Science*, 212:81–83.
23. Drenick, E. J. (1976): Weight reduction by prolonged fasting. In: *Obesity in Perspective, Fogarty International Center, Series on Preventive Medicine*, edited by G. A. Bray, pp. 341–360. D.H.E.W. Publication No. (N.I.H.) 75-708.
24. Drenick, E., Bales, G. S., Seltzer, F., and Johnson, D. G. (1980): Excessive mortality and causes of death in morbidly obese men. *JAMA*, 243:443–445.
25. Dwyer, J. (1980): Sixteen popular diets. Brief nutritional analyses. In: *Obesity*, edited by A. J. Stunkard, pp. 276–291. W. B. Saunders, Philadelphia.
26. Fain, J. N., and Shepherd, R. E. (1979): Hormonal regulation of lipolysis: Role of cyclic nucleotides adenosine and free fatty acids. *Adv. Exp. Med. Biol.*, 111:43–77.
27. Ferguson, J. M. (1976): *Habits, Not Diets*. Bull Publishing, Palo Alto.
28. Garrow, J. S. (1978): *Energy Balance and Obesity in Man*, 2nd edition. Elsevier, North-Holland Biomedical Press, Amsterdam.
29. Genuth, S. M., Castro, J. H., and Vertes, V. (1974): Weight reduction in obesity by outpatient semistarvation. *JAMA*, 230:987–991.
29a. Genuth, S. M. (1979): In: *Advances in Obesity Research*, edited by G. A. Bray.
30. Glick, Z., Teague, R. J., and Bray, G. A. (1981): Brown adipose tissue mediates the thermic effect of a single meal. *Science*, 213:1125–1127.
31. Gordon, E. S., Goldberg, M., and Chosy, G. J. (1963): A new concept in the treatment of obesity. *JAMA*, 186:156–166.
32. Government Printing Office. *Nutrition and your Health, Dietary Guidelines for Americans*.
33. Greenway, F. L., and Bray, G. A. (1977): Human chorionic gonadotropin (HCG) in the treatment of obesity: A critical assessment of the Simeons method. *West. J. Med.*, 127:461–463.
34. Greenway, F. L., Heber, D., and Bray, G. A. (1981): Failure of oral glycerol treatment to induce weight loss in obese humans. *Curr. Therap. Res.*, 29:849–852.
35. Gwinup, G. (1975): Effect of exercise alone on the weight of obese women. *Arch. Int. Med.*, 135:676–680.

36. Hirsch, J., and Batchelor, B. (1976): Adipose tissue cellularity in human obesity. *Clin. Endocrinol. Metab.*, 5:299–311.
37. Howard, A. N. (1979): Possible complications of long-term dietary treatment of obesity. In: *Medical Complications of Obesity: Proceedings of the Serono Symposia, Vol. 26*, edited by M. Mancini, B. Lewis, and F. Contaldo, pp. 349–363. Academic Press, London.
38. Howard, A. N., editor (1981): *Symposium on the use of very low calorie diets. Int. J. Obes.*, 5:193–352.
39. Innes, J., Campbell, I. W., Campbell, C. J., Needle, A. L., and Munro, J. F. (1974): Long term follow-up of therapeutic starvation. *Br. Med. J.*, 2:356–359.
40. Jordan, H. A., Levitz, L. S., and Kimbrell, G. M. (1976): *Eating is Okay. A Radical Approach to Successful Weight Loss. The behavioral control diet explained in full.* Edited by Steve Gelman, Rawson Associated Publishers, Inc., New York.
41. Kinsell, L. W., Gunning, B., Michaels, G. D., Richardson, J., Cox, S. E., and Lemon, C. (1964): Calories do count. *Metabolism*, 13:195–204.
42. Kissileff, H. R., Pi-Sunyer, F. X., Thornton, J., and Smith, G. P. (1981): C-terminal octapeptide of cholecystokinin decreases food intake in man. *Am. J. Clin. Nutr.*, 34:154–160.
43. Knittle, J. L., Timmers, K., Ginsberg-Fellner, F., Brown, R. E., and Katz, D. P. (1979): The growth of adipose tissue in children and adolescents. Cross-sectional and longitudinal studies of adipose cell number and size. *J. Clin. Invest.*, 63:239–246.
44. Pilkington, T. R. E., Gainsborough, H., Rosenoer, V. M., and Carey, M. (1960): Diet and weight reduction in the obese. *Lancet*, 1:856.
45. Porte, D., and Woods, S. C. (1981): Regulation of food intake and body weight by insulin. *Diabetologia*, 20:274–279.
46. *Recommended Dietary Allowances* (1980): National Academy of Sciences. Washington, D.C., 9th Rev. Ed.
47. Rodin, J., Bray, G. A., Atkinson, R. L., Dahms, W. T., Greenway, F. L., Hamilton, K., and Molitch, M. (1977): Predictors of successful weight loss in an out-patient obesity clinic. *Int. J. Obes.*, 1:79–87.
48. Rodin, J. (1981): Psychological factors in obesity. In: *Recent Advances in Obesity Research: III. Proceedings of the Third International Congress on Obesity*, edited by P. Bjorntorp, M. Cirella, and A. N. Howard, pp. 106–123. John Libbey, London.
49. Schachter, S., and Rodin, J. (1974): *Obese humans and rats*, edited by L. Festinger and S. Schachter, Lawrence Erlbaum Assoc., Potomac.
50. Scoville, B. (1976): Review of amphetamine-like drugs by the Food and Drug Administration: Clinical data and value judgments. In: *Obesity in Perspective. A conference sponsored by the John E. Fogarty International Center for Advanced Study in the Health Sciences*, edited by G. A. Bray, pp. 441–443. D.H.E.W. Publication No (N.I.H.) 75–708.
51. Sours, H. E., Frattali, V. P., Brand, D., Feldman, A. L., Swanson, R. C., and Paris, A. L. (1981): Sudden death associated with very low calorie weight reduction regimens. *Am. J. Clin. Nutr.*, 34:453–461.
52. Stein, M. R., Julis, R. E., Peck, C. C., Hinshaw, W., Sawich, J. E., and Diller, J. J., Jr. (1976): Ineffectiveness of human chorionic gonadotropin in weight reduction. A double-blind study. *Am. J. Clin. Nutr.*, 29:940–948.
53. Stuart, R. B., and Davis, B. (1972): *Slim Chance in a Fat World: Behavioral Control of Obesity.* Research Press Co., Champaign.
54. Stunkard, A. J., and McLaren-Hume, M. (1959): The results of treatment for obesity. *Arch. Intern. Med.*, 103:79–85.
55. Sullivan, A. C., and Comai, K. (1978): Pharmacological treatment of obesity. *Int. J. Obes.*, 2:167–189.
56. Wing, R. R., and Jeffrey, R. W. (1979): Outpatient treatments of obesity: A comparison of methodology and clinical results. *Int. J. Obes.*, 3:261–279.
57. Yang, M. U., and Van Itallie, T. B. (1976): Composition of weight lost during short-term weight reduction. *J. Clin. Invest.*, 58:722–730.
58. Young, C. M., Hutter, L. F., Scanlan, S. S., Rand, C. E., Lutwak, L., and Simka, V. (1972): Metabolic effects of meal frequency in normal young men. *J. Am. Diet Assoc.*, 61:391–398.
59. Young, C. M., Scanlan, S. S., Im, H. S., and Lutwak, L. (1971): Effect on body composition and other parameters in obese young men of carbohydrate level of reduction diet. *Am. J. Clin. Nutr.*, 24:290–296.

Health and Obesity, edited by H. L. Conn, Jr.,
E. A. DeFelice, and P. Kuo. Raven Press,
New York © 1983.

Behavior Therapy and Obesity

Albert J. Stunkard and Thomas A. Wadden

*Department of Psychiatry, University of Pennsylvania School of Medicine,
Philadelphia, Pennsylvania 19104*

Psychological factors have long been accorded an important place in the treatment of obesity. Adherence to dietary instructions has been recognized as an essential element of treatment, and intuitively based efforts at improving adherence, ranging from psychological support to scare tactics, have been utilized by clinicians for more than one-half a century. Particularly since the rise of psychoanalysis, more theoretically-based efforts have been utilized in an attempt to deal with such putative causes of overeating as orality, anxiety reduction, or just simple boredom. Most of the efforts have been unsystematic and unevaluated.

More systematic approaches to treatment have been introduced in recent years, including hypnosis (44), supportive psychotherapy (51), self-help groups (2,43), and psychoanalysis (29,38). By far the best studied and most thoroughly evaluated psychological therapy, however, has been behavior modification.

Interest in behavior modification began in 1967 with the publication of a short paper, "Behavioral Control of Overeating" (33). This interest rapidly developed into a virtual explosion of research, and reports of 150 clinical trials have made obesity the single most thoroughly researched topic in behavior therapy and perhaps in all of psychotherapy research.

In this chapter we review some major characteristics of behavior therapy, the results of behavior therapy of obesity, and, in some detail, a recent study that has demonstrated the superiority of behavior therapy to pharmacotherapy in the treatment of overweight adults. We then describe two important applications of behavioral weight control—its promising but still largely unexplored use with children and its widespread but only partially successful use in self-help programs. The chapter closes with a description of the major components of a behavioral weight control program.

SOME MAJOR CHARACTERISTICS OF BEHAVIOR THERAPY

Behavior therapy of obesity has often been equated with tricks or gimmicks—such as laying down one's fork between bites, pausing during the course of a meal, or using distinctive table settings. As such, it appears to fill a need for something new and different for those people who are constantly preoccupied with their weight and how to control it. As useful as some of these tricks or gimmicks may be, this view of behavior therapy does a serious disservice to attempts to understand the field. It confuses specific tactics with a system of therapy and, perhaps more important, a distinctive way of looking at human behavior (or more broadly, at human nature). Behavior therapy, or its equivalent, behavior modification, is derived from a set of assumptions that extends directly back to the radical behaviorism of John B. Watson and, less directly, to the nominalist schoolmen of the Middle Ages. Although it developed out of the systematic application of experimentally derived principles of learning to the modification of problem behaviors, behavior therapy has extended far beyond its origins, so that today it enjoys no generally accepted definition. Nevertheless, a series of core characteristics convey a sense of the boundaries of this new and rapidly developing field (49).

The first of these core characteristics is the assumption that all behavior, normal and abnormal, is acquired and maintained according to definable principles, many of which are already known. A second characteristic is one that contrasts strongly with those of other psychological systems. It is that people are best described by their behavior—what they think, feel, and do in specific situations—not by dispositional tendencies such as hostility and insecurity. A third characteristic of behavior therapy is the attempt to specify treatment measures as precisely as possible and to evaluate outcomes by the most objective possible measures. Behavior therapists have been in the forefront of efforts to introduce treatment manuals of even greater specificity and to evaluate outcomes in the patient's environment. For example, they were the first to assess the efficacy of treatments for phobias by observation of patients in the phobic situation.

A fourth characteristic of behavior therapy is the individualization of treatment. Although this characteristic is not peculiar to behavior therapy, it is important to mention it as a corrective to some popular views that equate behavior therapy with a kind of "Clockwork Orange" disregard of individuality in the single-minded pursuit of behavior change. Similarly, the goals of treatment are set by negotiation between the patient and therapist, and they are renegotiated at periodic intervals. Finally, every effort is made to provide continuing and critical assessment of treatment throughout its course.

THE RESULTS OF BEHAVIOR THERAPY OF OBESITY

A large number of studies have shown that behavior therapy is more effective than a variety of alternate treatments for mild and moderate obesity (37). But, this demonstration, although well established, tells us little about the effectiveness of behavior therapy as a practical measure for the control of obesity. Furthermore, several factors make it difficult to obtain a clear picture of the clinical impact of behavior therapy of obesity. Many studies of treatment have been conducted by inexperienced therapists in nonclinical settings, and over short periods of time. Most of the subjects have been mildly overweight college students rather than clinically obese patients, and far too many of the studies have been content with ascertaining the relative effectiveness of small differences in technique.

Despite these problems in assessment, definitive findings have emerged, and a review of 21 recent reports provides a basis for judging the overall efficacy of behavioral treatment for obesity. Six important issues will be examined before considering the all-important issue of weight loss.

(a) The first important finding is that considerable progress has been made in decreasing dropouts from treatment. Whereas dropouts from traditional out-patient treatment were as high as 25 to 75% (37) most behavioral programs report rates of 15% or less (47). A well-controlled trial has confirmed the widespread clinical impression that contingency contracting, or the earning back of deposits made by patients at the beginning of treatment, is very effective in decreasing dropouts (16).

(b) A second major advance has been in the reduction of untoward side effects of weight loss regimens, a problem that has plagued routine medical office treatment of obesity. As many as one-half of all obese patients undergoing such treatment may suffer from such symptoms as anxiety, irritability, and depression (42). By contrast, untoward reactions to behavioral programs are uncommon.

(c) There is great variability in weight change during treatment and even greater variability following treatment. Wilson notes that this variability suggests that the critical factors governing weight loss have not been identified or that current behavioral methods are appropriate only for persons with some still undetermined characteristics (47).

(d) Prediction of the outcome of behavioral treatments for obesity has not been very successful, and only a few relatively weak predictors have been discovered. This failing is particularly troubling in view of the marked variability in treatment outcome. If outcome could be predicted more accurately, more effective use could be made of scarce treatment resources, and many patients would be spared the time, effort, and discouragement of still another experience of failure.

(e) Patients with onset of obesity early in life lose as much weight as those with onset in adult life (17). This finding appears somewhat at variance with predictions based on expected fat cell size and number.

(f) Despite the fact that behavioral techniques can be adapted for use by less skilled therapists, skill of the therapist appears to have a modest effect on outcome of therapy. Two studies have shown that therapist experience was positively related to weight loss (17,20).

Weight Loss During Treatment

The most important measure of treatment efficacy is weight loss. Wing and Jeffery's (50) review of the literature on the treatment of obesity during the preceding decade reveals that weight losses produced by behavior therapy do not differ greatly from those produced by other forms of treatment and that none of these therapies is particularly effective. Figure 1 shows that behavior therapy and pharmacotherapy contributed the largest number of studies. In each, the average weight loss was no more than 5.1 kg.

A more detailed analysis of the behavioral programs was presented by Jeffery et al. (17), who confined their review to 21 reports that met basic criteria for adequacy

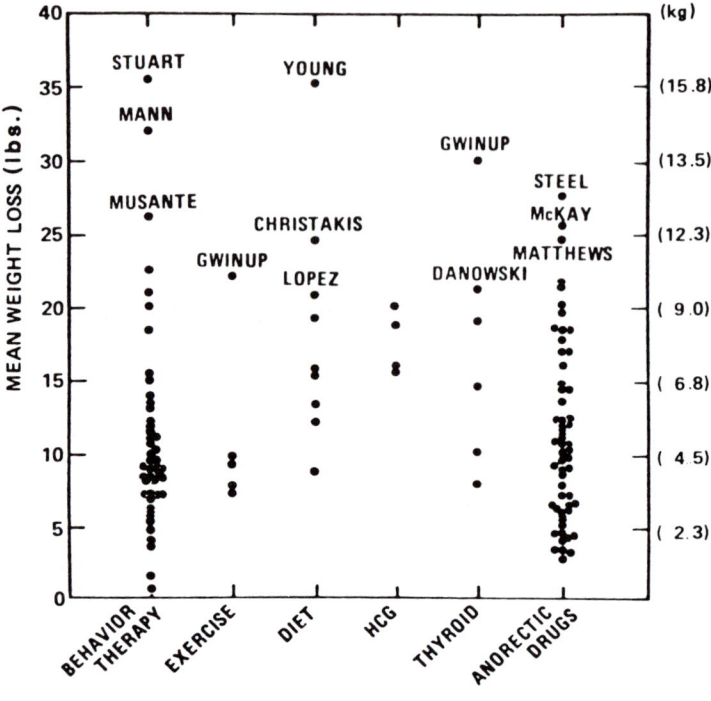

FIG. 1. Distribution of weight losses in studies of outpatient therapy for obesity. (From Wing and Jeffery, ref. 50, with permission.)

of research design. These criteria included basing the results on all patients who started treatment (including dropouts) and reporting weight losses in pounds rather than simply in percentage of excess weight. Table 1 shows that weight losses of no more than one-half the programs exceeded 4.5 kg and losses of only 20% exceeded 6.8 kg. There are many reasons for these limitations—most of the programs were short term, many involved patients who were only mildly overweight, and a large number were carried out by inexperienced therapists. But the fact remains: the results are modest and, from the perspective of clinical utility, disappointing. Furthermore, progress is hard to see; no study has even equaled the results of the original 1967 report that ignited the explosion of interest in the behavioral control of obesity.

These results from the research literature are not dissimilar to those from a program with a primarily clinical focus. Jeffery et al. (17) found a weight loss of no more than 5.0 kg among the first 125 patients in a behaviorally oriented obesity treatment program.

Maintenance of Weight Loss

Investigators working in the late 1960s believed that behavior therapy would promote long-term maintenance of weight loss and that patients would even continue

TABLE 1. *Results of behavioral treatments for obesity[a]*

Study	n	Initial weight (kg)	Mean weight loss[b] (kg)	Treatment length (weeks)
Abrams and Allen (1974)	23	83.0	5.4	9
Hagen (1974)	18	69.5	6.8	10
Hall (1972)	10	78.6	1.5	4
Hall et al. (1974)	40	—	5.0	10
Hall et al. (1975)	25	89.8	6.8[c]	12
Hanson et al. (1976)	32	96.4	5.9[c]	10
Harris (1969)	7	77.8	3.1	10
Harris and Bruner (1971)	11	74.9	3.4	12
Harris and Bruner (1971)	6	65.3	.8	16
Harris and Hallbauer (1973)	27	75.2	3.6	12
Jeffery (1974)	34	83.5	2.7	7
Levitz and Stunkard (1974)	73	82.2	1.9	12
Mahoney (1974)	9	—	3.4	8
McReynolds (1976)	41	81.1	7.9	15
Penick et al. (1971)	15	114.1	10.1	12
Romanczyk (1974)	17	79.9	4.8	6
Romanczyk et al. (1973)	18	81.3	3.2	4
Romanczyk et al. (1973)	18	78.6	3.6	4
Stuart (1967)	8	83.4	17.2	52
Stuart (1971)	6	—	6.4	15
Wollersheim (1970)	18	70.0	4.7	12

[a]From Jeffery et al. (17).
[b]Data describe the most effective treatment combination only. Results from control groups and partial treatments are not included.
[c]Extrapolated from weight reduction indices.

to lose weight after treatment had concluded. These hopes have only been partially realized. In their review of 17 controlled studies with a 1-year follow-up, Wilson and Brownell (48) found almost no change in mean weight loss from posttreatment ($\bar{x}$ = 4.72 kg) to follow-up ($\bar{x}$ = 4.64 kg). Stunkard and Penick, (41) reviewing 10 studies that overlapped somewhat with the 17 of Wilson and Brownell (48), interpreted the results less optimistically, noting that maintenance of weight loss occurred primarily when the losses were not clinically significant. Even in the few studies in which clinically significant weight losses appeared to be maintained, they may not have been! Stunkard and Penick (28, 41) reported the largest weight loss (9.6 kg) and the best apparent maintenance (a further 2.5 kg lost) in a controlled trial of behavior therapy. This apparent maintenance, however, was actually a statistical artifact resulting from a loss of weight following treatment by many patients who had lost little weight during treatment. Those who had lost weight during treatment tended to regain it. The correlation between weight change during treatment and follow-up was actually a negative one (-0.499, $p < 0.10$).

It appears that weight losses achieved with behavior modification are, at best, modestly maintained, and only a handful of studies have shown weight loss after treatment ended (41,48). The effectiveness of behavioral programs in achieving long-term weight reduction would best be assessed by comparison with the results of other treatments. Until recently, however, such a comparison was not possible because comparable data from other kinds of treatment were not available. This situation has been corrected by a recent investigation by Craighead et al. (12). The study, the largest controlled trial of behavior therapy of obesity, is worth describing in some detail.

BEHAVIOR THERAPY AND PHARMACOTHERAPY OF OBESITY

This investigation was undertaken to determine the relative effectiveness of behavior therapy and pharmacotherapy, the two leading treatments of obesity. It assessed the effects of behavior therapy alone, pharmacotherapy (fenfluramine) alone, and the combination of the two therapies in 98 obese women during 6 months of treatment and at a 1-year follow-up. There were three major treatments and two control groups.

(a) Behavior therapy was presented in a highly structured program that utilized Ferguson's manual (13) and modifications of the Mahoneys' book (23).

(b) Pharmacotherapy consisted of fenfluramine in doses up to 120 mg/day, as tolerated, with tapering of dosage during the last month of treatment. In addition, patients received supportive group counseling designed to reproduce the nonspecific elements of the behavior therapy condition.

(c) Combined treatment included both behavior therapy as described for the first condition, and fenfluramine, as prescribed by resident physicians in the second condition.

(d) The doctor's office medication control group was designed to approximate traditional office treatment for obesity. It was composed of patients of resident physicians who provided traditional medical treatment, including medication (fenfluramine), a reducing diet, instructions for exercise, and advice and encouragement. After 6 months, they were given additional treatment in groups and so were not included in the follow-up.

(e) The waiting list control group patients were assessed, placed on a waiting list, weighed at 4 and 6 months, and then provided treatment. They were also not included in the follow-up.

Patients in the three major treatment conditions met weekly for 6 months in groups of 10 for 1½ hr. Two female therapists, one a doctoral and one a master's level clinical psychologist, each led two 10-person groups in each of the three major treatment conditions—a total of 12 groups. Resident physicians were responsible for administration of the fenfluramine.

Patients consisted of 98 obese women who were 63% overweight, whose median age was 47, and who were over middle socioeconomic status. They were randomly assigned from stratified blocks (based on percentage overweight) to treatment conditions, as follows: behavior therapy, 32; pharmacotherapy, 25; combined treatment, 23; doctor's office control, 8; waiting list control, 10.

Weight Loss

The patients in all treatment groups lost significantly more weight than those in the waiting list control group, who gained 1.3 ± 1.3 kg ($p < 0.001$; Fig. 2). The weight losses of the pharmacotherapy (14.5 ± 1.1 kg) and combined treatment patients (15.3 ± 1.2 kg) did not differ significantly and both were significantly greater than the weight losses of the behavior therapy patients (10.9 ± 2.0 kg, $p < 0.05$).

Patients in the physician's office medication control group lost only 6.0 ± 1.7 kg, significantly less than the 14.5 ± 1.1 kg lost by the pharmacotherapy patients ($p < 0.05$). The drug dosage in the two groups was the same; only the circumstances of its administration differed.

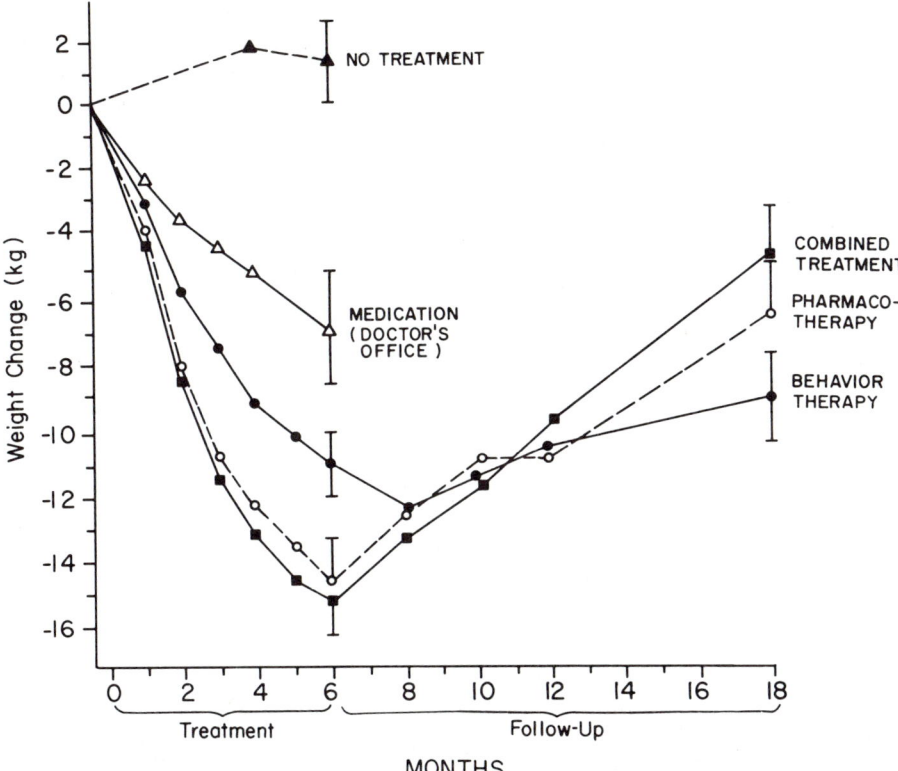

FIG. 2. Weight changes during 6 months of treatment and 12 months of follow-up. The three major treatment groups lost large amounts of weight during treatment: behavior therapy *(solid circles)* 10.9 kg, pharmacotherapy *(open circles)* 14.5 kg, and combined treatment *(solid squares)* 15.3 kg. Behavior therapy group continued to lose weight for 2 months and then slowly regained it, in contrast to rapid regain of weight by pharmacotherapy and combined treatment groups. Among the control groups, the no-treatment *(solid triangles)* control group gained weight, whereas the doctor's office *(open triangles)* medication group lost 6.0 kg. Patients in these two groups received additional treatment at 6 months and so were not available for follow-up. Vertical lines represent 1 SEM. (From Craighead et al., ref. 12, with permission.)

The results of the 1-year follow-up of 100% of the patients in the three major treatment conditions showed a striking reversal in the relative efficacy of the treatments. Far less weight was regained by behavior therapy patients than by pharmacotherapy and combined treatment patients ($p < 0.001$). In fact, behavior therapy patients continued to lose weight during the first 2 months of follow-up and at 1 year had regained only 1.9 ± 1.0 kg, for a net weight loss from the beginning of treatment of 9.0 ± 1.3 kg. By contrast, pharmacotherapy patients regained 8.2 ± 1.2 kg, for a net loss of only 6.3 ± 1.5 kg. Combined treatment patients regained even more weight (10.7 ± 1.2 kg) than pharmacotherapy patients, for an even smaller net weight loss (4.6 ± 1.6 kg). The resulting trend in net weight loss favored behavior therapy alone over the two conditions that utilized pharmacotherapy [F (2.72) = 2.82, p < 0.07].

Although fenfluramine, administered in a group setting, produced significantly greater weight loss than did behavior therapy, this benefit was short-lived. Patients who had received fenfluramine regained weight far more rapidly following treatment than did those who received only behavior therapy. This poor maintenance of weight loss soon erased any advantage of pharmacotherapy. One year after treatment, patients who had received only behavior therapy showed a net weight loss greater than those who had received medication. Furthermore, adding fenfluramine to behavior modification not only did not improve the long-term results, it compromised them. The long-term results were actually poorer among behavior therapy patients who had also received fenfluramine than among those who had not.

It is not clear how the addition of medication compromised the long-term effects of behavior therapy. There are at least two possible explanations, one psychological and one pharmacological. A psychological explanation derives from attribution theory in general and from Bandura's theory of self-efficacy in particular (3, 4). These theories suggest that patients who received combined treatment may have attributed their weight loss to the pharmacological intervention rather than to their own efforts in changing behavior. If so, they would have failed to develop the increased sense of self-efficacy that should accompany increased behavioral self-control. Therefore, when their pharmacological support was withdrawn, releasing biological pressures to regain weight, their undeveloped sense of efficacy would have provided little assistance. Interviews at the 1-year follow-up supported this interpretation. By contrast, patients who received only behavior therapy attributed their weight loss to their own efforts. The increased sense of self-efficacy apparently strengthened their efforts at controlling their weight. Just such consequences of self-efficacy attributions were demonstrated in a small-scale study by Chambliss and Murray (10).

In terms of the pharmacological explanation, the most likely cause is that fenfluramine lowered a body weight set point, thereby facilitating weight loss. Discontinuation of fenfluramine permitted the set point to return to its pretreatment level. The resulting biological pressures to gain weight to this higher level produced weight gains of greater magnitude than those of patients who had lost weight without pharmacological aid (39).

The study showed in a dramatic manner how the circumstances of its administration may influence medication. Administered in a traditional doctor's office format, fenfluramine produced a weight loss of 6.0 kg, a bit more than is customary in routine clinical practice. Slightly altering the circumstances of its administration (group meeting with the use of a deposit to encourage attendance) more than doubled this loss, from 6.0 kg to 14.5 kg. Furthermore, this altered format showed a highly favorable cost-effectiveness ratio. Far less professional time was spent with each patient than in the traditional one-to-one format.

The results of this study cast serious doubt on the widely held belief that tolerance develops to the effects of appetite-suppressant medication (39). The usual clinical criterion for the development of tolerance is the slowing of the rate of weight loss during the course of treatment. By this criterion, the minimal slowing of weight loss in the pharmacotherapy condition suggests that tolerance did not develop.

Even slowing of weight loss is probably not an adequate criterion of tolerance. Slowing of weight loss occurs in all forms of treatment for obesity, and a recent review has described at least four causes other than tolerance (39). A better measure of tolerance is failure to regain weight after treatment. Also by this criterion, tolerance did not develop. Weight was regained rapidly after medication was stopped. Apparently fenfluramine had continued to be effective.

Maintenance of the therapeutic effectiveness of fenfluramine for as long as 6 months has important policy implications. Current restrictions on the long-term use of appetite suppressants are based in large part on the belief that patients become tolerant to the effects of such medication. If tolerance does not develop, these restrictions are less reasonable and long-term pharmacotherapy for obesity becomes more plausible.

BEHAVIORAL WEIGHT CONTROL FOR CHILDREN

The studies reviewed thus far (as most of the research on behavioral weight control) have involved the treatment of obese adults. Until recently, by contrast, the problems of childhood obesity have been largely unexplored. The results of the few well-controlled studies with children are promising. They are described briefly here, as is, in more detail, an innovative program involving the use of parents in the treatment of overweight adolescents.

Behavior therapy for obese children was first shown to be more effective than no treatment by Wheeler and Hess (46) in a study of 40 overweight children, aged 2 to 11. The children were randomly assigned to one of two conditions. In the behavioral condition, children and parents met in individual one-half hr sessions every 2 weeks for an undisclosed period, and then less frequently as they "made progress." They undertook a carefully specified regimen (36) that included record keeping, stimulus control, and reinforcement. Children in a control condition received no treatment.

Six children dropped out of each condition, and 14 subjects remained. Those children remaining in the behavioral group decreased their average percentage overweight from 40 to 35%, whereas those remaining in the control group increased their average percentage overweight from 39 to 44%. Although this difference was said to be statistically significant, the results are difficult to interpret because of the disparity in age among the subjects, the absence of data on actual weight loss, and the lack of follow-up.

In a more elaborate study by Weiss (45), 47 children (11 boys, 36 girls), aged 9 to 18 and averaging 42.6% overweight, were assigned to one of five treatment conditions:

(a) Diet, no reward—children were given an exchange diet and were awarded points for following the diet. The points were not exchanged for reinforcers.

(b) Diet, self-reward—the same exchange diet was used, and the children earned points that they exchanged for self-administered reinforcers such as watching television.

(c) Stimulus control—cue control behaviors were prescribed.

(d) Stimulus control, diet, self-reward—combination of conditions, a, b, and c.

(e) No-treatment control.

Subjects were seen individually for 12 weekly sessions of 10 to 15 min each. Parents of all children were merely instructed "not to interfere."

Fourteen of the 47 subjects dropped out of treatment, leaving 33 participants. After 12 weeks, subjects in the behavioral groups lost significantly more weight (0.3 to 1.3 kg) than the no-treatment control group (a gain of 1.9 kg). The treatment groups did not differ significantly. At 1-year follow-up, the children in the two stimulus control groups (c and d) had performed significantly better (-0.1 and $+0.7$ kg) than those in the other three groups, who had gained 4.3 kg (diet, no reward), 3.5 kg (diet, self-reward), and 8.2 kg (no-treatment).

Although these two studies demonstrated that behavior therapy is better than no therapy, they left many questions unanswered, one of which was how important is parental influence.

Since parents play a critical role in their child's obesity (25), it seems reasonable that they might also play an important role in its treatment. Two groups have assessed this role by including parents as active members in treatment programs for their obese children. The first study showed only a trend for the parents to facilitate weight loss; the second study showed a strong effect.

Kingsley and Shapiro (19) studied the influence of parental participation in the treatment of 24 boys and 16 girls, aged 10 and 11, from relatively affluent families. The children were randomly assigned to one of four conditions:

(a) Child only—children attended treatment sessions alone and were instructed in recording food intake and stimulus control behaviors.

(b) Mother only—mothers attended meetings alone and learned procedures identical to those in the child only condition.

(c) Mother and child together—children and mothers attended all meetings together and received the program described above.

(d) Waiting list control—treatment was deferred for 8 weeks.

Treatment sessions occurred weekly for 8 weeks. A $30 deposit could be earned back by attending all sessions.

Children in the three treatment groups lost significantly more weight (1.6 kg) during the 8-week program than did those in the no-treatment control group (who gained an average of 0.9 kg). The three treatment conditions, however, did not differ from each other during or after treatment. During follow-up, children who had been in the treatment groups gained an average of 0.4 kg per month, approximately the expected developmental weight gain. Those in the mother-child together group had regained less weight at follow-up, but the difference between this and the other groups did not reach statistical significance, perhaps because of the small sample size and the large variance in weight losses.

Brownell et al. (9) conducted a study similar to Kingsley and Shapiro's. The investigation was carried out with 42 children (33 girls and 9 boys), who averaged 55.7% overweight and 13.8 years of age. Three treatment conditions were assessed.

(a) Mother-child separately—mothers and children each attended sessions, but met concurrently in separate groups. Children were instructed in behavioral techniques of weight control, as detailed in a treatment manual (7). Mothers were told that they were crucial to their children's success and were instructed in ways of facilitating weight reduction. Mothers and children were encouraged to discuss their feelings about obesity and dieting, to share their family experiences, and to work together in a spirit of cooperation.

(b) Mother-child together—the mothers and children attended all treatment sessions together and met in the same groups. They were told that this was a useful approach because the mothers and children would understand one another, would profit from hearing the others in the group, and would be able to practice the program components together. Aside from the difference in parent involvement, children received the same treatment program as described above.

(c) Child alone—the children met in groups, but the mothers did not participate in the formal treatment. The children were encouraged to share the materials from the treatment manual with their parents, but were told that they would do best if they could learn to control their eating on their own. The basic treatment program was otherwise the same as that used for the other two groups.

In all treatment conditions, meetings lasted for 45 to 60 min and were held in groups of 5 to 8 participants. A total of 16 weekly sessions were provided.

Changes in percentage overweight are presented in Fig. 3. At the end of treatment, the change in percentage overweight for the mother-child separately condition (-17.1%) was significantly greater than the change for the mother-child together (-7%) and child-alone (-6.8%) conditions. Figure 4 shows the weight loss for the mother-child separately condition was 8.4 kg, compared to 5.3 kg, and 3.3 kg for the mother-child together and child-alone conditions, respectively.

The superiority of the mother-child separately condition was even more pronounced at 1-year follow-up, as shown in Fig. 3. Although the mother-child together

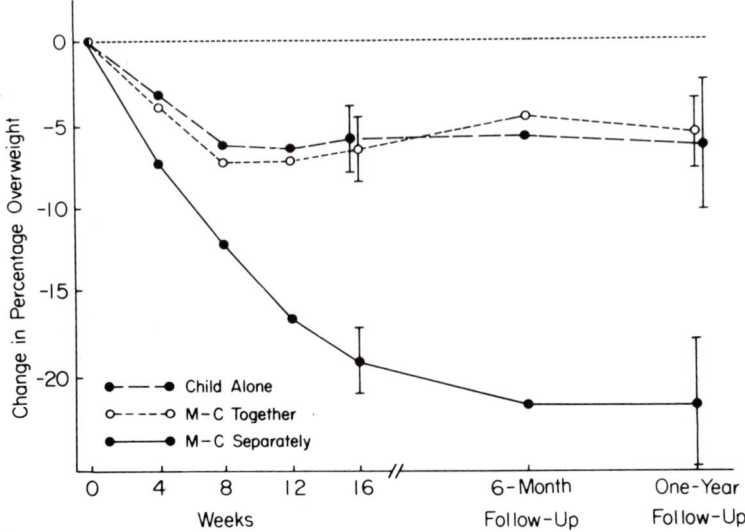

FIG. 3. Changes in percentage overweight after 16 weeks of treatment and at 6- and 12-month follow-up. Subjects in the mother-child (M-C) separately condition achieved a significantly greater decrease in percentage overweight, at all assessment periods, than subjects in the child alone and mother-child (M-C) together conditions. (From Brownell et al., ref. 9, with permission.)

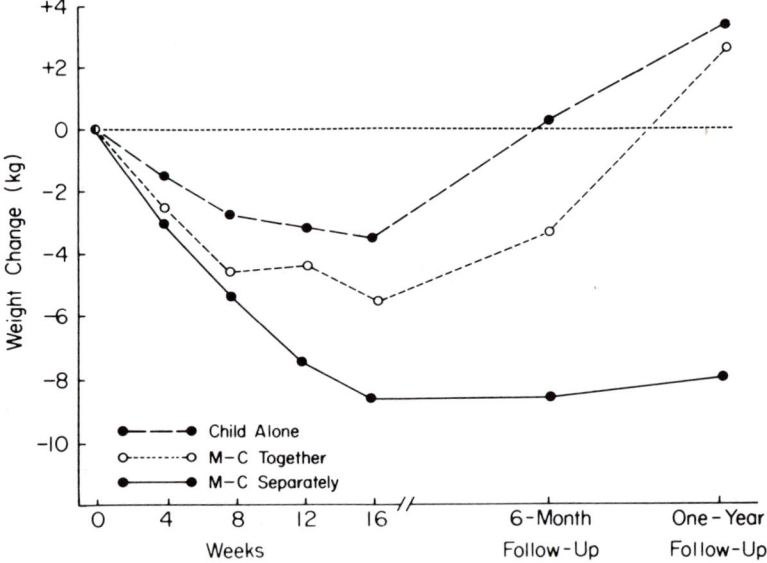

FIG. 4. Weight change (in kg) for child alone, mother-child (M-C) together, and mother-child (M-C) separately conditions after 16 weeks of treatment and 6- and 12-month follow-up. (From Brownell et al., ref. 9, with permission).

and child-alone conditions had maintained their decreases in percentage overweight (-5.5% and -6%, respectively), the mother-child separately group had decreased even further (-20.5%).

In terms of absolute weight change at the 1-year follow-up, children in the mother-child separately condition (-7.7 kg) again weighed significantly less than those in the mother-child together and child-alone conditions. Children in both of these groups had actually gained approximately 3 kg over their pretreatment weight.

It should be noted that children in these latter two groups maintained the decrease in their degree of obesity during follow-up, despite the gain in weight. Increased weight was offset by increased height so that there was no change in percentage overweight.

There are several possible reasons for the greater weight losses in the mother-child separately group. First, children in the child-alone group did not attend well to the therapist and were prone to disruptive behavior. The mothers' involvement in the other two groups seemed to make the children more responsive to the therapist. Second, mothers and children in the mother-child together group were reluctant to voice negative feelings about the problems of dealing with the other. The mother-child separately group allowed both parties to discuss sensitive issues. These findings are consistent with the predictions one would make from developmental psychology. Adolescents face the difficult task of seeking independence from the parents on whom they are financially and emotionally dependent (39). Too much independence (child-alone group) may create aggressive reactions because of the lack of structure, and too much parental involvement (mother-child together group) may not give the child the necessary sense of responsibility. It appears, therefore, that treating mothers and children separately has the advantages of: (a) providing training for both parents and children, (b) allowing free discussion by both parents and children, and (c) making the children more responsible and better controlled than if the parents do not participate.

THE WIDESPREAD APPLICABILITY OF BEHAVIORAL TECHNIQUES

The encouraging results of behavioral treatment achieved in the Craighead et al. (12) study have revived a flagging interest in the application of behavioral techniques to the treatment of mild and moderate obesity. There is every likelihood that further research may produce still further increases in therapeutic efficacy. But small, incremental advances in the improvement of clinical practice ignore what may well be the major contribution of behavioral technology to the control of obesity—its applicability to large groups.

One of the most important aspects of behavioral technology is that it can be precisely specified and, thus, can be easily taught and learned, even by persons with less than a professional education. Indeed, a revealing finding of the early study by Penick et al. (28) was that the behavior therapy program was carried out by a team with little experience in the modality or in the treatment of obesity and, yet, it was more effective than the best alternative program of a highly skilled treatment team. In fact, the inexperienced behavior therapists achieved a twofold increase in weight loss over experienced conventional therapists. Lesser increases in effectiveness have brought about major changes in the management of other disorders. The question arises—can the precise specification of behavioral techniques permit their application to populations larger than the clinical ones for which they were developed?

The answer is "yes." Behavioral therapy has been widely applied in self-help treatments for obesity, and today more obese people are receiving such treatment than are receiving medical attention for it. For example, one-half million people a week receive behavior therapy for obesity under the auspices of just one commercial weight reduction program—Weight Watchers.

SELF-HELP PROGRAMS AND BEHAVIOR THERAPY

In this section we discuss the nature and efficacy of self-help programs and the application of behavior therapy to them. The two most popular self-help programs, TOPS (Take Off Pounds Sensibly) and Weight Watchers, share several similarities. Both hold weekly meetings, lasting approximately 1½ hr, at which members officially weigh in and then participate in a group support effort. Successful dieters are praised for their accomplishments, and those who have failed during the week are encouraged not to give up trying.

Participants in both programs pay an initial registration fee ($13 for Weight Watchers). Thereafter, members of TOPS, a nonprofit organization, pay an annual fee of approximately $10, whereas members of the commercially operated Weight Watchers are charged $5 per week. Weight Watchers members who meet their goal weight are eligible to attend monthly classes without charge for life, provided that they remain within 2 pounds of their goal weight and do not miss a monthly meeting. For persons who can meet these rigid requirements, this contractual agreement is a powerful incentive for maintenance of weight loss.

Weight Watchers introduced three significant changes in the basic TOPS format (40). First, a palatable, satisfying, and well-balanced diet has been designed by nutritional experts and is marketed in many commercial outlets. Although more expensive than comparable food bought in grocery stores, the controlled portion size facilitates dietary adherence and contributes to the effectiveness of the program for that minority of members who use these packaged foods. Second, weekly talks are given by a paid lecturer who provides basic information about the program. Lecturers are selected from among persons who have successfully completed the Weight Watchers program, and they are often highly effective speakers, possessed of charismatic qualities. Third, a program of behavior modification has been introduced into Weight Watchers.

How effective are these programs? Considerable information is available about TOPS, which, from time to time, has permitted persons outside the organization to investigate its performance. The average TOPS member is a 42-year-old woman with an ideal weight (calculated from standard height-weight tables) of 54.1 kg.

She enters TOPS weighing 85.5 kg, which is 31.4 kg or 58% over her ideal weight. She stays in TOPS for 16½ months and loses 6.8 kg (40).

Although these results are impressive for an organization that costs little and makes few demands on its membership, they almost certainly overestimate the efficacy of treatment. The reason for this overestimation is the pattern of membership in TOPS. The organization is characterized by a high dropout rate. Studies have revealed that approximately one-half of the members of any TOPS group drop out of it within 1 year, and by the end of the second year, more than two-thirds have dropped out (40). Membership in TOPS at any given time appears to consist of a relatively small group of long-term members and a larger pool of those who have been in the organization for only a short time (14).

The high dropout rate is not attributable to members who achieved a significant weight loss and then leave satisfied. On the contrary, the high attrition rate is due to dissatisfaction with the program and with the failure to lose weight. The pattern of weight loss of members who remain in TOPS for longer periods of time is of interest. Apparently they lose a significant amount of weight early in their membership. Thereafter, they stop losing weight and begin to regain it. The optimist can view such a record as favorable—relatively effective maintenance of weight loss is achieved—an uncommon occurrence in the management of obesity. The pessimist might focus on the majority of patients who lose little weight and drop out of the program.

For the clinician, self-help groups provide an all-too-often neglected resource for the care of patients. Only 6% of the members of TOPS are referred by their physicians (40). Given their low cost, benign character, and favorable results— even if for only a minority—self-help groups for obesity should be considered by all physicians who treat obese persons. Furthermore, knowing that dropping out of these groups constitutes a major problem, and that staying in the groups is often associated with modest success, the physicians can educate patients about these facts and use their influence to encourage remaining in the program.

The high attrition rates of self-help groups probably constitute the major barrier to their effectiveness. Since one of the principal contributions of behavior therapy to the treatment of obesity has been its ability to reduce attrition and improve adherence to therapeutic regimens, a combination of self-help and behavior therapy seemed to offer a promising "therapeutic coalition for obesity" (20). This strategy was tested by Levitz and Stunkard (20) in a large-scale clinical trial that enrolled 234 members of TOPS. Four treatment conditions were applied to each of four chapters. Treatments included: (a) behavior therapy conducted by a professional therapist; (b) the same program conducted by a TOPS chapter leader; (c) nutrition education provided by the TOPS leader; and (d) continuation of the usual TOPS program.

Behavior therapy increased the effectiveness of the TOPS program, sharply reducing the attrition rate and increasing weight loss. During the 3 months of active treatment, fewer TOPS members dropped out of the two behavioral interventions than out of the nutrition education and control groups. At 9 months follow-up, this difference had become striking. Only 38 and 41% had dropped out of the behavior therapy groups, compared with 55 and 67% for the nutrition education and control groups respectively (Fig. 5).

These differential attrition rates biased the results against behavior therapy, for decreased attrition means retaining less successful members. Nonetheless, the behavioral programs produced significantly greater weight losses than the control treatments. TOPS chapters in which behavior therapy was conducted by a professional therapist lost 1.9 kg, which was significantly more than the reductions in the nutritional education (-0.1 kg) or the TOPS control group (in which subjects actually gained 0.3 kg). Professional therapists using the behavioral program produced significantly greater losses than TOPS chapter leaders using the same interventions (-1.9 kg versus -0.9 kg).

Differences between groups had increased at a 9-month follow-up (Fig. 6). Subjects in the professionally conducted behavior therapy program increased their weight loss to 2.6 kg. The initial weight loss of subjects in the behavioral intervention conducted by TOPS chapter leaders was not maintained, with the subjects' weight returning to pretreatment levels. However, these individuals had better results than subjects in the nutrition education and control conditions, who gained weight during follow-up (1.3 and 1.8 kg, respectively).

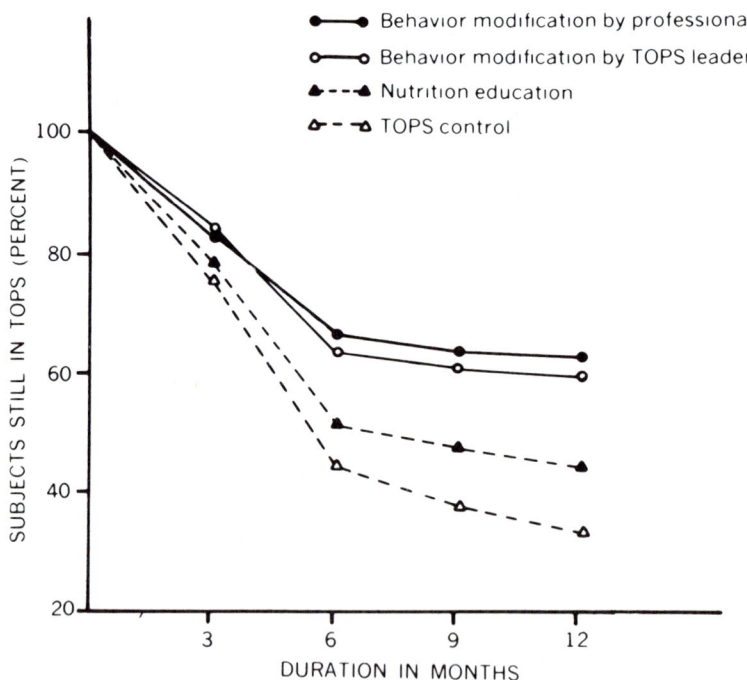

FIG. 5. Attrition rate of TOPS subjects over a 1-year period under four experimental conditions. (From Levitz and Stunkard, ref. 20, with permission).

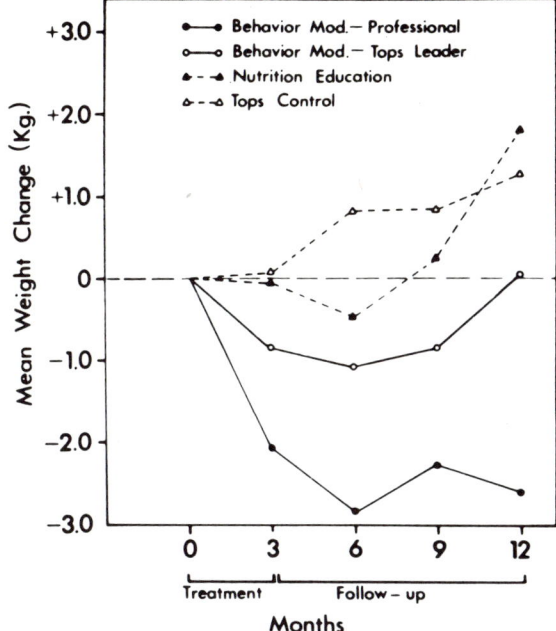

FIG. 6. Weight changes (in kg) of TOPS subjects over a 1-year period under four experimental conditions. (From Levitz and Stunkard, ref. 20, with permission.)

The results of this investigation, modest as they were, demonstrated that behavior therapy could significantly improve the effectiveness of TOPS, particularly by alleviating its major problem—attrition. One might have thought that TOPS would have eagerly exploited this finding to which it had made such an important contribution. Curiously, it has shown no such inclination, and the chief beneficiaries have been TOPS' competitors—the commercial weight reduction programs.

The largest of the commercial weight reduction programs, Weight Watchers, added a sophisticated behavioral program to its traditional measures of inspirational lectures, group pressure, and diet. The first report of this new program indicates that it improved performance (34). Weight losses, which had averaged 0.5 kg per week under the traditional program increased to 0.6 kg per week with the addition of behavior therapy.

This increase in weight loss is gratifying and further supports the value of adding a behavioral component to traditional self-help programs for obesity. Weight Watchers, however, has not released information concerning the effects of the behavioral intervention on the far more serious problem of attrition rates. A recent report, however, suggests that high attrition continues to plague these organizations. Volkmar et al. (43) studied 108 women enrolled in a commercial weight reduction program that purported to include a strong behavioral component. In two experimental conditions, subjects who also received the standard program were rewarded for weight loss according to two different schedules of reinforcement; in the control condition, subjects received only the standard program. Figure 7 shows that very high attrition rates occurred in all three treatment conditions—50% of the subjects had dropped out of the program at 6 weeks and 70% at 12 weeks. The fact that such high attrition occurred among persons who were receiving the standard treatment, as well as those in the two experimental conditions, suggests that marked attrition may be a consistent feature of these programs. This suggestion is corroborated by a review of the literature on the attrition rates in commercial weight reduction groups.

The only other prospective study is that of Nash (27), who reported dropout rates remarkably similar to those of the study by Volkmar et al. (43). She found that persons joining the group had previously joined and dropped out an average of three times and that the more often persons joined, the more likely they were to drop out.

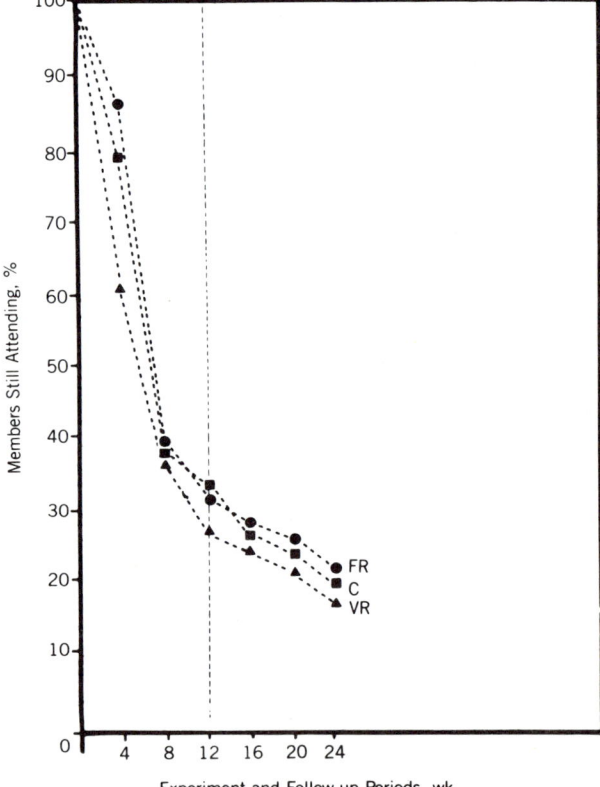

FIG. 7. Life table of subjects remaining under observation for 24 weeks, showing dropout rates during experimental and follow-up periods. During the first 12 weeks, subjects received experimental treatment plus standard treatment; during the second 12 weeks, they received only standard treatment. FR represents fixed ratio schedule; VR, variable ratio schedule; and C, control. (From Volkmar et al., ref. 43, with permission.)

The results of the studies by Nash (27) and Volkmar et al. (43) are represented in Fig. 8, together with those of four retrospective studies reported by Ashwell (1). These latter four studies were conducted on a Weight Watchers group in Australia and three British groups—Weight Watchers, Silhouette Slimming Clubs, and Slimming Magazine Slimming Clubs. The most notable aspects of all these reports is the similarity in the attrition rates in programs with different procedures and different samples, conducted on three continents.

These findings underscore the fact that reports of self-help groups for obesity must be regarded with great caution, for they must clearly be based on a very select sample of persons. Those dropping out of treatment are usually persons with the smallest weight losses and reports based only on treatment "survivors" will consequently be highly biased. Any cross-sectional assessment of treatment results may produce inflated weight losses due to the dropout of less successful members. Valid estimates of the weight losses achieved by self-help groups can only be obtained

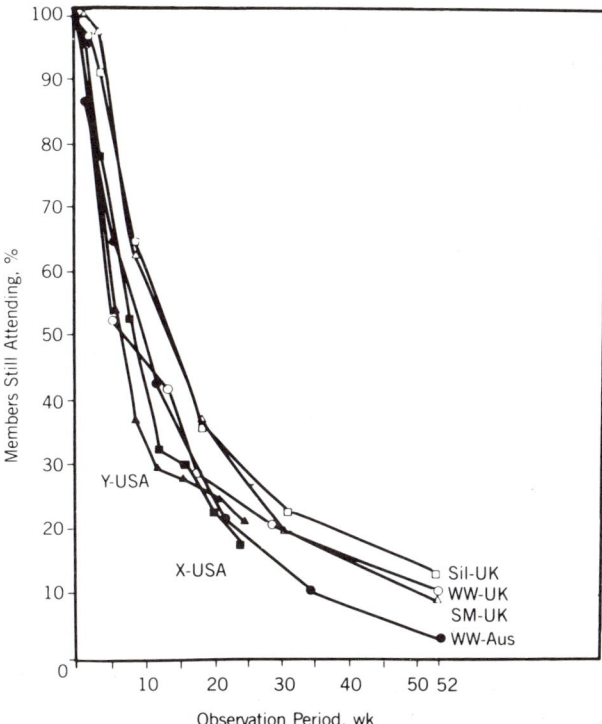

FIG. 8. Life table of participants in six treatment programs under observation for up to 52 weeks, showing dropout rates during first year of membership. Data from Nash (27) is depicted as X-USA and from Volkmar et al. (43) as Y-USA. The four studies reported by Ashwell (1) represent: Silhouette Slimming Club, United Kingdom (Sil-UK); Weight Watchers, United Kingdom (WW-UK); Slimming Magazine, United Kingdom (SM-UK); and Weight Watchers, Australia (WW-Aus) (as recalculated, assuming that subjects not responding to questionnaire had dropped out of treatment). (From Volkmar et al., ref. 43, with permission.)

through cohort studies that consider all persons entering a program and their weight change at the time they leave it.

DESCRIPTION OF A BEHAVIORAL PROGRAM

In this section we provide a description of the behavioral program for weight control. A detailed report is beyond the limits of this chapter, and the interested reader is referred to the extended descriptions of Mahoney and Mahoney (23), Jordan et al. (18), and Stuart (35) and to the manuals by Ferguson (13). Nevertheless, a brief description of some of the essential elements may be useful. Measures to increase physical activity and provide nutrition education are important components, but we will focus here on five more explicit behavioral measures designed to control food intake. Four have been elements of most behavioral programs; the fifth is increasingly utilized in these programs: (a) Self-monitoring—description of the behavior to be controlled; (b) control of the stimuli that precede eating; (c) development of techniques to control the act of eating; (d) reinforcement of the prescribed behaviors; and (e) cognitive restructuring.

(a) Self-monitoring—description of the behavior to be controlled. Patients are asked to keep careful records of the food they eat. Each time they eat, they write down precisely what it was, how much, at what time of day, where they were, who they were with, and how they felt. The immediate reaction of many patients to this time-consuming and inconvenient procedure is grumbling and complaints. Such reactions occurred far more frequently in the early days of these programs and may well have been due to the therapists' own uncertainty about the technique. More recently, patients have responded more positively. Many come to the view that record-keeping may be the single most important part of the behavioral program. It vastly increases patients' awareness of their eating behavior. Despite their years of struggle with the problem, once patients begin to keep records, they are surprised at how much they eat and how varied are the circumstances in which they eat.

There is a surprising unanimity on the value of self-monitoring. It is true that some have found the effects rather weak (24,32) or of limited duration (22,36). Others, however, report robust effects (6,15,30,31). The more specific the items monitored, the more effective the results. Not only is self-monitoring a key element in the process of behavior change, it is the mainstay of the behavioral assessment of obesity (8).

(b) Control of the stimuli that precede eating. A behavioral analysis traditionally begins with a study of the events antecedent to the behavior to be controlled. Stimulus control of eating involves many kinds of measures that are traditional in weight-reduction programs. For example, every effort is made to limit the amount of high-calorie food kept in the house and to limit accessibility to food that must be kept in the house. For times when eating cannot be resisted, adequate amounts of low-calorie foods, such as celery and raw carrots, are kept readily available.

In addition, behavioral programs introduced new and distinctive measures. For example, most patients reported that their eating took place in a wide variety of places and at many different times during the day. Some note that, if they eat while watching television, it is not long before watching television makes them eat. It is as if the various times and places had become discriminative stimuli for eating. In an effort to decrease the number and potency of discriminative stimuli that control their eating, patients are encouraged to confine all eating, including snacking, to one place. In order not to disrupt domestic routines, this place is very frequently the kitchen.

A parallel effort is made to develop new discriminative stimuli for eating and to increase their power. For example, patients are encouraged to use distinctive table settings, perhaps an unusually colored placemat and napkin, and special silver. No effort is made to decrease the amount of food patients eat, but they are encouraged to use the distinctive table settings whenever they eat, even for a small between meals snack. One middle-aged housewife, convinced of the importance of this measure, went so far as to take her distinctive table setting with her whenever she dined out. She was an early success.

Stimulus control has occupied a central position in most behavioral weight control programs of the past decade, but its independent contribution to the efficacy of these programs is not known. Only two studies have attempted to assess this efficacy by comparing stimulus control alone to other treatment modalities and they have reached opposite conclusions. McReynolds et al. (26) reported that stimulus control alone was as effective as a treatment package that contained it, whereas Loro et al. (21) found stimulus control alone "to be a relatively ineffective weight-loss procedure." This latter study, it should be noted, involved weight losses of only 2.7 and 3.2 kg even in the relatively more effective weight-loss procedures. Stimulus control appears sufficiently useful to continue as a major element in behavioral programs despite the sparsity of controlled evidence for its independent efficacy. Its efficacy is likely to be considerably increased if it is used specifically for persons in whom pretreatment behavioral assessment has revealed deficiencies in this area (11).

(c) Development of techniques to control the act of eating. Specific techniques are utilized to help patients decrease their speed of eating, become aware of all the components of the eating process, and gain control over these components. Exercises include counting each mouthful of food eaten during a meal or each chew or each swallow. Patients are encouraged to practice putting down their eating utensils after every third mouthful until that mouthful is chewed and swallowed. Then longer delays are introduced, starting with 1 min toward the end of the meal when it is more easily tolerated, and moving to more frequent delays, longer ones, and ones earlier in the meal.

Patients are encouraged to stop pairing their eating with such activities as reading the newspaper and watching television, and to make conscious efforts to make eating a pure experience. They are urged to do whatever they can to make meals a time of comfort and relaxation, particularly to avoid old arguments and new problems at the dinner table. They are encouraged to savor the food as they eat it, to make a conscious effort to become aware of it as they are chewing, and to enjoy the act of swallowing and the warmth and fullness in their stomachs. To the extent that they succeed in this endeavor, they eat less and enjoy it more.

(d) Reinforcement of the prescribed behaviors. In addition to the informal and incidental rewards that patients receive from the behavioral program, a system of formal rewards is also used. Separating the reward schedules for changes in behavior and for weight loss is useful; rewards for changing behavior may be the more effective.

In order to decrease the time between the exercise of a specific behavior and the attendant reward, patients are awarded a certain number of points for each of the activities that they are learning: record-keeping, counting chews and swallows, pausing during the meal, eating in one place, and so forth. Not only do patients receive a certain number of points for each activity, but they can earn extras, such as double the number of points, when they devise an alternative to eating in the face of strong temptation.

These points, which serve to provide immediate reinforcement of a behavior, are cumulated and converted into more tangible rewards, often in concert with the spouse. Popular rewards include a trip to the movies or relief from housekeeping chores. A more impersonal reward is conversion of points into money, which patients bring to the next meeting and donate to the group. Surprisingly altruistic courses may be chosen. In an early program, one group donated its savings to the Salvation Army, another to a needy friend of one of the members.

Promptness of the reinforcement seems a key to success. One middle-aged house-wife said, "My husband was always offering to buy me a car if I lost 50 pounds. I used to work away at it and knock myself out and lost 30 pounds, which was a lot of weight, but what did it get me? I didn't get half a car. I got nothing. I've only lost eight pounds in this program so far and he's done all sorts of good things for me."

(e) Cognitive restructuring. In the quite recent past, behavior therapy has been enriched by an interest in cognitions and by the new field of cognitive-behavior modification. Concern with cognitions has received less attention in the treatment of obesity than have more traditional operant concerns, and there has been as yet only limited experimental evidence for the efficacy of cognitive strategies in the treatment of obesity. Nevertheless, these strategies have been attracting increasing attention and several clinicians believe that they can make a useful contribution to an overall program of treatment for obesity.

A feature that has made cognitions palatable to the more behavioristic therapists is recognition that the internal monologues that occupy so much of our time are readily accessible. Furthermore, they can be quantified and treated very much as any traditional operant in terms of reinforcement, extinction and so forth. Mahoney and Mahoney (23) have directed attention to the critical role that cognitions and private monologues may play in the maintenance and control of obesity. The first step in applying cognitive strategies to weight control is to help patients discover their most common negative monologues, or self-statements, and to estimate their frequency. Then, in the manner described by Beck (5), patients are taught arguments against these monologues. Since negative monologues tend to be stereotyped and limited in number, it is usually not difficult to construct arguments against them. The patient is then helped to learn—and overlearn—these more appropriate self-statements so that they can use them almost automatically in response to the negative statements. Training in this kind of arguing with oneself seems to produce benefits in terms of improved morale, as has been shown quite convincingly in the case of depression, and probably also in more effective weight-reducing behaviors. Simply repeating the counterarguments over a period of time may help; even if the person does not completely believe them at the onset.

In their description of "cleaning up the cognitive ecology," the Mahoneys (23) describe five kinds of negative self-statements. Examples from my experience, together with counterarguments are:

Weight loss: "It's taking so long to lose weight." A counterargument is, "But I am losing it. And this time I'm going to learn how to keep it off."

Ability to lose weight: "I've never done it before. Why should I succeed this time?" A counterargument is, "There always has to be a first time. And this time I've got a good new program going for me."

Goals: "I've got to stop snacking!" A counterargument is "That is an unrealistic goal. Just keep on trying to cut down the number of snacks."

Food thoughts: "I keep finding myself thinking how good chocolate tastes." A useful response is, "Stop that! It's just frustrating you. Think of lying on the beach in the sun" (or whatever activity the patient finds particularly enjoyable).

Excuses: "Everyone in my family has a weight problem. It's in my genes." A counterargument is, "That just makes it harder, not impossible. If I stick with this problem, I will succeed."

SUMMARY AND CONCLUSIONS

The large experimental and clinical literature on behavior therapy of obesity that has appeared in the 15 years since its introduction permits a confident assessment of behavior therapy's current status and future prospects. It is important to recognize that behavior therapy of obesity consists of far more than the tricks and gimmicks with which it is usually associated. It constitutes, rather, a system of therapy based on a strong experimental tradition and a distinctive way of looking at human behavior. It has been responsible for notable advances in treatment—decreasing dropouts and reducing untoward psychological responses. It has not, however, achieved large weight losses, and the losses that it has produced have been only partially maintained. A recent study, however, has given grounds for some optimism regarding the future. Clinically significant weight losses (10.9 kg) were achieved in a large number of obese women, and these weight losses were maintained far more effectively than those achieved by drug therapy (12).

Behavior therapy is just beginning to be applied to the treatment of childhood obesity, and a recent study suggests that it may have a bright future. Treating obese children concurrently with the treatment of their mothers appeared to optimize the results.

The mechanics of behavior therapy can be precisely specified and easily taught and learned. It has, therefore, been possible to introduce behavioral treatment into self-help groups for obesity, and, today, more people are receiving behavior therapy for obesity under lay auspices than are receiving medical attention for it. Very high dropout rates and a paucity of unbiased reports from these organizations make it difficult to assess the value of these efforts. Those persons who persist in behavior therapy provided under lay auspices probably achieve considerable benefit, and referral of patients to such groups is a reasonable option for the practicing physician.

We conclude that behavior therapy for obesity is a well-established and modestly effective treatment for mild to moderate obesity. It is safe and well accepted, and, particularly in its application through lay self-help groups, available to very large numbers of persons who might otherwise have little access to treatment. The application of behavior therapy to childhood obesity is in its infancy and shows great promise. The most important aspect of behavior therapy, however, is its strong experimental tradition. This tradition makes it likely that we can look forward to continuing progress in the behavior therapy of obesity.

REFERENCES

1. Ashwell, M. (1978): Commercial weight loss groups. In: *Recent Advances in Obesity Research: II*, edited by G. Bray, pp. 266–276. Newman Publishing Co., London.
2. Ashwell, M., and Garrow, J. S. (1975): A survey of three slimming and weight control organizations in the U.K. *Nutrition*, 29:346–356.
3. Bandura, A. (1977): Self-efficacy: Toward a unifying theory of behavioral change. *Psychol. Rev.*, 84:191–215.
4. Bandura, A. (1978): Self-efficacy: Toward a unified theory of behavioral change. *Adv. Behav. Res. Ther.*, 1:139–161.
5. Beck, A. T. (1976): *Cognitive Therapy and the Emotional Disorders.* International Universities Press, New York.
6. Bellack, A. S., Rozensky, R., and Schwartz, J. S. (1974): A comparison of two forms of self-monitoring in a behavioral weight reduction program. *Behav. Ther.*, 5:523–530.
7. Brownell, K. D. (1979): *Behavior Therapy for Weight Control: A Treatment Manual.* Unpublished manuscript, University of Pennsylvania.
8. Brownell, K. D. (1981): Assessment of eating disorders. In: *Behavioral Assessment of Adult Disorders*, edited by D. Barlow, pp. 329–404. Guilford Press, New York.
9. Brownell, K. D., Kelman, S. J., and Stunkard, A. J. (1981): *The Role of Parental Participation in the Treatment of Obese Adolescents.* Manuscript submitted for publication, University of Pennsylvania.
10. Chambliss, C. A., and Murray, E. J. (1979): Efficacy attribution, locus of control, and weight loss. *Cognitive Ther. Res.*, 3:349–353.
11. Coates, T. J. (1977): *The Efficacy of a Multi-Component Self-Control Program in Modifying the Eating Habits and Weight of Three Obese Adolescents.* Published doctoral dissertation, Stanford University. Berkeley, California.
12. Craighead, L. W., Stunkard, A. J., and O'Brien, R. M. (1981): Behavior therapy and pharmacotherapy for obesity. *Arch. Gen. Psychiatry*, 38:763–768.
13. Ferguson, J. M. (1975): *Learning to Eat: Leaders Manual and Patients Manual.* Bull Publishing Co., Palo Alto.
14. Garb, A. R., and Stunkard, A. J. (1974): Effectiveness of a self-help group in obesity control. *Arch. Intern. Med.*, 134:716–720.
15. Green, L. (1978): Temporal and stimulus factors in self-monitoring by obese persons. *Behav. Ther.*, 9:328–341.
16. Hagen, R. L., Foreyt, J. P., and Durham, T. W. (1976): The dropout problem: Reducing attrition in obesity research. *Behav. Ther.*, 7:463–471.

17. Jeffery, R. W., Wing, R. R., and Stunkard, A. J. (1978): Behavioral treatment of obesity: The state of the art in 1976. *Behav. Ther.*, 9:189–199.
18. Jordan, A. H., Levitz, L. S., and Kimbrell, G. M. (1976): *Eating Is Okay.* Rawson, New York.
19. Kingsley, R. G., and Shapiro, J. (1977): A comparison of three behavioral programs for control of obesity in children. *Behav. Ther.*, 8:30–36.
20. Levitz, L. S., and Stunkard, A. J. (1974): A therapeutic coalition for obesity: Behavior modification and patient self-help. *Am. J. Psychiatry*, 131:423–427.
21. Loro, A. D., Fisher, E. B., and Levenkron, J. C. (1979): Comparison of established and innovative weight-reduction treatment procedures. *J. Appl. Behav. Anal.*, 12:141–155.
22. Mahoney, M. J. (1974): Self-reward and self-monitoring techniques for weight control. *Behav. Ther.*, 5:48–57.
23. Mahoney, M. J., and Mahoney, K. (1976): *Permanent Weight Control.* W. W. Norton, New York.
24. Mahoney, M. J., Mouro, N. G., and Wade, T. C. (1973): The relative efficacy of self-reward, self-punishment, and self-monitoring for weight loss. *J. Consult. Clin. Psychol.*, 40:404–407.
25. Mayer, J. (1968): *Overweight: Causes, Cost, and Control.* Prentice-Hall, Englewood Cliffs.
26. McReynolds, W. T., Lutz, R. N., Paulsen, B. K., and Kohrs, M. B. (1976): Weight loss resulting from two behavior modification procedures with nutritionists as therapists. *Behav. Ther.*, 7:283–291.
27. Nash, J. D. (1977): *Curbing Drop-out from Treatment for Obesity.* Unpublished doctoral dissertation, Stanford University.
28. Penick, S. B., Filion, R., Fox, S., and Stunkard, A. J. (1971): Behavior modification in the treatment of obesity. *Psychosom. Med.*, 33:49–55.
29. Rand, C. S. W., and Stunkard, A. J. (1978): Obesity and psychoanalysis. *Am. J. Psychiatry*, 135:547–551.
30. Romanczyk, R. G. (1974): Self-monitoring in the treatment of obesity: Parameters of reactivity. *Behav. Ther.*, 5:531–540.
31. Romanczyk, R. G., Tracey, D. A., Wilson, G. T., and Thorpe, G. L. (1973): Behavioral techniques in the treatment of obesity: A comparative analysis. *Behav. Res. Ther.*, 11:629–640.
32. Stollack, G. E. (1967): Weight loss obtained under different experimental procedures. *Psychotherapy: Theory, Research, Practice.* 4:61–64.
33. Stuart, R. B. (1967): Behavioral control of overeating. *Behav. Res. Ther.*, 5:357–365.
34. Stuart, R. B. (1977): Self-help for self-management. In: *Behavioral Self-Management*, edited by R. B. Stuart, pp. 278–305. Brunner/Mazel, New York.
35. Stuart, R. B. (1978): *Act Thin, Stay Thin.* W. W. Norton, New York.
36. Stuart, R. B., and Davis, B. (1972): *Slim Chance in a Fat World: Behavioral Control of Obesity.* Research Press, Champaign.
37. Stunkard, A. J. (1975): From explanation to action in psychosomatic medicine: The case of obesity. *Psychosom. Med.*, 37:195–236.
38. Stunkard, A. J. (1980): Psychoanalysis and psychotherapy. In: *Obesity*, edited by A. J. Stunkard, pp. 355–368. W. B. Saunders, Philadelphia.
39. Stunkard, A. J. (1981): Anorectic agents: A theory of action and lack of tolerance in a clinical trial. In: *Anorectic Agents: Mechanisms of Action and Tolerance*, edited by S. Garattini and R. Saminin, pp. 191–210. Raven Press, New York.
40. Stunkard, A. J., Levine, H., and Fox, S. (1970): The management of obesity: Patient self-help and medical management. *Arch. Intern. Med.*, 125:1067–1072.
41. Stunkard, A. J., and Penick, S. B. (1979): Behavior modification in the treatment of obesity. The problem of maintaining weight loss. *Arch. Gen. Psychiatry*, 36:801–806.
42. Stunkard, A. J., and Rush, J. (1974): Dieting and depression reexamined. A critical review of reports of untoward responses during weight reduction for obesity. *Ann. Intern. Med.*, 81:526–533.
43. Volkmar, F. R., Stunkard, A. J., Woolston, J., and Bailey, R. A. (1981): High attrition rates in commercial weight reduction programs. *Arch. Intern. Med.*, 141:426–428.
44. Wadden, T. A., and Flaxman, J. (1981): Hypnosis and weight loss: A preliminary study. *Int. J. Clin. Exp. Hypnosis*, 29:162–173.
45. Weiss, A. R. (1977): A behavioral approach to the treatment of adolescent obesity. *Behav. Ther.*, 8:720–726.
46. Wheeler, M. E., and Hess, K. W. (1976): Treatment of juvenile obesity by successive approximation control of eating. *J. Behav. Ther. Exper. Psych.*, 7:235–241.

47. Wilson, G. T. (1980): Behavioral modification and the treatment of obesity. In: *Obesity*, edited by A. J. Stunkard, pp. 325–344. W. B. Saunders, Philadelphia.
48. Wilson, G. T., and Brownell, K. D. (1980): Behavior therapy for obesity: An evaluation of treatment outcome. *Adv. Behav. Res. Ther.*, 3:49–86.
49. Wilson, G. T., and O'Leary, K. D. (1980): *Principles of Behavior Therapy*. Prentice-Hall, Englewood Cliffs.
50. Wing, R. R., and Jeffery, R. W. (1979): Outpatient treatments of obesity: A comparison of methodological and clinical results. *Int. J. Obes.*, 3:261–272.
51. Wollersheim, J. P. (1970): Effectiveness of group therapy based on learning principles in the treatment of overweight women. *J. Abn. Psych.*, 76:462–274.

Health and Obesity, edited by H. L. Conn, Jr., E. A. DeFelice, and P. Kuo. Raven Press, New York © 1983.

Fasting and Modified Fast Diets in Treatment of Obesity

Victor Vertes

Department of Medicine, Mount Sinai Medical Center, Cleveland, Ohio 44106

There is little disagreement that the best approach to weight reduction is the conventional low calorie diet (1,000 calories) coupled with increased caloric expenditure. Theoretically, this should be the logical mode of treatment. In practice, however, despite concentrated efforts, few patients can maintain themselves on this approach long enough to effect any significant progress. Stunkard and McLaren-Hume (17) reported that as few as 5% of patients under conventional outpatient care could lose 18 kg (40 lb) or more and only 25% were able to lose as much as 9 kg (20 lb). For the massively obese, those who weigh 100% or more of their ideal body weight, this certainly does not offer a viable choice.

Surgical approaches include jejunoileal bypass and gastric stapling. The former procedure has proven, for the most part, unsatisfactory in the majority of cases. Mortality rates have been estimated at 3% (5). Morbidity is virtually 100%, with weakness, hypokalemia, and diarrhea the most common side effects. Gastric stapling is a new and, perhaps, exciting surgical approach. It has a much lower mortality rate associated with the operation itself and the morbidity is decreased. This may be a viable option for a select group of massively obese patients when less invasive procedures have failed.

In our experience the only medical approach that has proven effective in the majority of the massively obese is the use of a modified fasting regimen. Fasting as a therapeutic tool has been known since the time of Hippocrates (13). Additionally, the ability of the human body to adjust to long periods of food deprivation has been utilized in religious fasting. Within this century political activists such as Mahatma Gandhi and, more recently, the IRA hunger strikers have chosen fasting as a means of protest.

The physiological effects of fasting are well known. After a 24 to 48 hr period, the patient will develop anorexia and often a mild state of euphoria. These positive effects, however, are balanced by a series of metabolic disorders. These include sodium loss, hypoglycemia, hyperuricemia, metabolic acidosis, hypokalemia, and, most importantly, a loss of lean body mass. This loss of lean body mass eventually leads to a cachectic state and can, if left untreated, end in death. This has been witnessed most recently with the protestors in Ireland where, predictably, death occurs after 50 to 70 days of fasting.

Fasting as an introduction to the treatment of obesity was proposed by Bloom (3) in the late 1950s. He observed that the weight loss of patients in full-fast was greater than could be explained by caloric deprivation. Short periods of starvation were well tolerated and effective.

Duncan et al. (7) demonstrated the use of intermittent fasting as a means of therapy for the intractably obese. Patients were hospitalized for from 5 to 14 days on a total fast. On discharge, patients were placed on a conventional diet (1,500 to 2,300 cal/day) for 6 days, followed by 1 to 2 day fasts. The regimen was continued at varying intervals to effect sustained weight reduction and to restrict the tendency to gain weight. Although this therapeutic approach was effective during the fasting period, it was an expensive method of treatment and applicable to only small groups of patients.

In the mid-1960s, Drenick et al. (6) demonstrated the feasibility of prolonged starvation in hospitalized patients. Patients were fasted for 12 to 117 days with weight losses of up to 52.6 kg (116 lb). As in the previous studies the patients tolerated the program easily. The major drawbacks of this study were the required hospitalization and cost. Although full fast does provide an approach to treatment of the massively obese, it is not without some serious problems. Mineral losses always accompany starvation. Natriuresis proceeds at either a uniformly low level or in a varying pattern that can lead to marked sodium depletion. Potassium deficiency usually develops, as do hyperuricemia, ketosis, and hypoglycemia. These findings are in addition to the serious problem of protein catabolism. Medical complications include severe orthostatic hypotension, gouty arthritis, and normocytic, normochromic anemia (Table 1).

Several investigators studied the importance of protein supplementation during periods of fasting in obese patients. Bolinger et al. (4) and Apfelbaum et al. (1) found that providing a small amount of exogenous protein during a short-term fast allowed for more favorable ratios of fat to nitrogen losses. This N-sparing effect was achieved without inhibiting the positive aspects of anorexia. Genuth (9) studied the effects of oral administration of the amino acid L-alanine on the group of fasting patients. He found that 50 gm of this major glucose precursor could counteract the metabolic complications of semistarvation. Muscle catabolism was reduced as measured by decreased plasma levels of essential branched chain amino acids and decreased urinary losses of phosphorus and potassium. Both hypoglycemia and hyperuricemia were lessened. This initial study was expanded into a program involving 75 patients on a supplemented modified fast diet composed of both protein and carbohydrate.

TABLE 1. *Effects of inadequate protein*

Decrease in lean body mass
Decreased resistance to infection
Decrease in work performance
Enzyme problems?

Following these early studies of semistarvation, three separate groups investigated the use of a modified fast in the treatment of the massively obese. Blackburn et al. (2) in Boston used small amounts of high biological value animal protein to maintain a positive nitrogen balance. Patients were carefully selected on the basis of nutritional history, individual dietary diaries, and Minnesota Multiphasic Personality Inventory. The initial study was begun with a period of hospitalization followed by outpatient care. The approach was later expanded to a total outpatient program. The investigators found that the protocol was well-tolerated, duplicated the beneficial effects of total starvation, and preserved lean body mass while maintaining nitrogen balance.

At the same time, Genuth et al. (11) in the United States and Howard and Baird (14) in England, independently, were judging the feasibility of a hypocaloric semisynthetic diet in the treatment of the massively obese. The study by Genuth et al. (11) involved 75 massively obese patients and demonstrated the success of a formula modified fast in achieving weight reduction without serious disabilities. The first 10 patients were hospitalized for 1 to 2 weeks at which time they were placed on a full fast. These patients were then given a supplement of casein and glucose during 1 more week of hospitalization. The subsequent 65 patients were placed on the supplement regimen immediately following completion of testing and were discharged from the hospital 1 week later. The protocol required weekly visits at which time the subjects were weighed, examined, and counseled. Blood chemistries were obtained at 1 to 3 week intervals. Results of this outpatient program were most encouraging. As contrasted with the 5% success rate reported by Stunkard and McLaren-Hume (17), 60% (47 patients) were able to lose 18 kg (40 lb) or more. The average weight loss was 38 kg (85 lb), with men losing at a higher rate than women. In addition to the marked clinical improvement of the patients, including increased exercise tolerance and a general sense of well-being, carefully monitored blood chemistries showed no significant abnormalities and no significant evidence of protein loss.

Other benefits of this approach included decreased blood pressure in the hypertensive patients; improvement of dyspnea, especially in those patients with complicating pulmonary or cardiac disease; relief of joint and/or back pain, increased exercise tolerance, and agility; and a sense of well-being and improved self-image. Along with the benefits, patients reported several common complaints. Although less than 10% of the subjects experienced these side effects, they included orthostatic hypotension, dizziness with rapid change of position, cold intolerance, transient erythematous rash, hair loss, dry skin, constipation, and halitosis (Table 2). Cholecystitis occurred in 2 patients after unsupervised realimentation. The success of the modified fast in effecting a substantial weight reduction was encouraging and led us to the development of a large-scale outpatient regimen (12). Of 519 patients, 78% lost 18 kg (40 lb) or more. The regimen was well accepted, allowed the patients to continue their normal activities, and caused no serious side effects. Howard and Baird (14) based their diet on egg albumin as the protein source. The diet regimen included the formula supplement, containing essential vitamins and

TABLE 2. *Symptoms—307 patients*
on Optifast®

	% of patients
Hair loss	9
Brittle nails	8
Dry skin	7
Cold intolerance	8
Muscle cramps	7
Tingling	7
Fecal impaction	0.6

minerals, and a safflower oil capsule. Noncaloric liquids were taken *ad libitum*. Like their American colleagues (2,11), Howard and Baird found that the degree of weight loss and compliance was greater than in conventional diets (800 to 1,000 kcal). Additionally, the patients received the same minimal daily requirements of vitamins, minerals, carbohydrates, and protein, as provided by the higher calorie conventional diets.

Although the original statistics of the pilot study of Genuth (9) were encouraging, the degree of success was tempered by the data from a survey taken 2 years later. Of the 47 patients (60% of the study) who had experienced successful weight reduction, 9% had stayed within 10% of their original weight loss, an additional 35% had regained less than one-half of the weight originally lost, and 56% had regained more than one-half of the weight (12). It became clear that, except for a small percentage of the massively obese population, a modified fast alone could be nothing more than another fad without an adequate follow-up program. At about the same time, reports of success in the treatment of obese patients by behavioral techniques were appearing in the literature (15). Although some degree of success utilizing these techniques alone could be achieved in moderate obesity, the results were at best poor in the massively obese. By combining the two approaches, supplemented fasting and behavioral techniques, the therapist can offer a potentially viable method of weight reduction to the massively obese patient (12,16).

We have come to view massive obesity as a chronic disorder of generally undetermined etiology. Cure of obesity, as defined by weight reduction followed by weight maintenance on an *ad libitum* intake, is rare. Control and palliation are more realistic approaches to treatment. We believe this therapy must have two phases: reduction and maintenance. This concept has been successfully instituted in our outpatient clinic (Table 3).

WEIGHT REDUCTION

Reduction, to be successful, must be done promptly and efficiently in a finite period of time. An understanding of proper patient selection is essential to the success of the supplemented fasting program. All patients are referred by their private physicians. A significant amount of weight needs to be lost (at least 50 lb);

TABLE 3. *Obesity is a chronic disorder*

Treatment: 2 phases
1. Reduction
    finite period of time
    fixed caloric intake
    maximum patient comfort
2. Maintenance
    behavior modification
    fixed and free caloric intake
    physical activity

this diet is too radical for minor weight reduction. Although some patients wishing relief solely from cosmetic and sociopsychological liabilities enroll in the program, the majority of patients have medical problems that can benefit from significant weight loss. Hypertension, adult-onset diabetes mellitus, and osteoarthritis all can be ameliorated. Patients are evaluated for intercurrent disease. Absolutely contraindicated for this regimen are advanced renal disease and hepatic failure, pregnancy or lactation, cerebrovascular disease, unstable angina, recent myocardial infarction, active deep vein thrombophlebitis, malignancy, active infective processes, treatment with chronic high dose steroids, and severe psychiatric problems with suicidal ideation. Age is also a contraindication; neither prepubertal nor geriatric subjects are accepted. Relative exclusions from the program include patients with a history of deep vein thrombosis, those involved in certain occupations, and those on specific psychotropic medication. Patient allergies also must be considered.

The protocol for the modified fast portion of our current program has remained essentially unchanged. Because the patients enter the program highly motivated, they are able to withdraw from food without much difficulty. We have found that the formula diet allows the necessary rapid, continuous weight loss while providing the patient with a no-choice, food-avoidance experience. The daily ration includes five portions of supplement containing protein and carbohydrate, a multivitamin tablet, and a potassium supplement when indicated. Noncaloric liquid should be taken *ad libitum*. All current medications are modified while a patient is on supplement. Diuretics and oral agents for diabetes mellitus are generally discontinued; insulin dosage is adjusted. Weekly clinic visits are required for weigh-in, counseling, and blood chemistries. A critical aspect of the regimen is the weekly lecture series, which presents information on nutrition, behavior modification, and physical activity. This introduction of new life skills is designed to facilitate long-term weight management (Table 4).

With careful patient selection, we have experienced no cardiovascular, renal, hepatic, or pulmonary problems. Early in the development of this program it was feared that deprivation of food, a central focus of their life, would cause acute depression in the patients. We found, however, no evidence of this. Quite the contrary is observed; euphoria at weight reduction seems to be the general tone of the clinic.

TABLE 4. *Nutrient composition of supplement*
Optifast®–70 per day

Protein	70 g	Magnesium	400 mg
Carbohydrate	30 g	Iron	18 mg
Sodium	40 mEq	Zinc	15 mg
Potassium	22 mEq	Manganese	4 mg
Calcium	1000 mg	Copper	2 mg
Phosphorus	550 mg	Calories	420

Our experience at Mt. Sinai Medical Center with this modified fast has been with more than 3,000 patients. Few medical complications have occurred. Two cases of cholecystitis and pancreatitis were reported immediately after improper self-realimentation. Five episodes of gout were recorded in 3 patients with a history of this disorder; no *de novo* attacks of gout were experienced. As with all diets in which a great deal of weight loss has occurred, there were several cases of reversible, unilateral peroneal nerve palsy caused by crossing of the legs. As a preventive measure, we caution our patients to sit with their legs uncrossed. We have recorded one case of a young woman, who, after great weight reduction, experienced a loss of self-identity. With professional help she was able to deal with the problem.

Unlike the data on liquid protein diets (8), we have had no unexplained sudden deaths in young females, age 25 to 44 years, the group designated as high risk. Our sudden death mortalities include one accidental death, four acute myocardial infarctions in patients with past histories of significant coronary and/or cardiovascular disease, and one death caused by subacute bacterial endocarditis.

The positive aspects of this mode of therapy are many. As previously stated, the modified fast generates a predictable weight loss, average rate of 1.4 kg (3 lb) per week for women and 2.0 kg (4.5 lb) per week for men. The weight loss proceeds in a linear fashion; the amount lost is closely correlated with the starting weight. Accompanying this decreased weight are the chemical benefits mentioned earlier.

Massive obesity is often associated with other medically complicating disorders including hypertension, adult-onset diabetes mellitus, high triglycerides, osteoarthritis, coronary disease, gallbladder disease, and Pickwickian syndrome. In a group of 99 hypertensive obese patients in our clinic, the effect of weight loss on diastolic pressure and need for medication was encouraging. Before modified fasting therapy, 47% of subjects were mildly hypertensive, with diastolic pressures of 90 to 99 mmHg; 32% had diastolic pressures of 100 to 109 mmHg; 21% had pressures greater than 110 mmHg. At the termination of therapy, 69% of patients had diastolic pressures less than 90 mmHg; 20%, 90 to 99 mmHg; 11%, greater than 100 mmHg. Whether this change in blood pressure is due to diuresis and sodium depletion or loss of body mass or a combination of the two is not clearly defined at the present time. Most patients entering this supplemented fasting program who are on hypertensive medication will tolerate withdrawal of their drugs. A small portion of this population will have to resume medication in spite of an acceptable weight loss.

Palliation of obesity yields improvements in diabetes mellitus, hyperinsulinism, and carbohydrate intolerance. In most instances those patients on oral agents of 45 units or less of insulin are able to discontinue their medication. Subjects taking more than 45 units of insulin follow a variable course, but generally decrease their insulin need. Other medically beneficial effects of this therapy include normalization of Type 4 electrophoretic patterns and high triglycerides. Improvement in dyspnea is noted, especially in patients with complicating pulmonary or cardiac disease. Loss of body mass has also enabled some patients to proceed with elective surgery.

Although not medical in nature, the social and cosmetic benefits of weight reduction must be considered. The sense of personal accomplishment, more favorable self-image, and greater acceptance by others are important aspects of the success of this program.

WEIGHT MAINTENANCE

Whereas acceptable weight reduction is the goal of phase one of obesity therapy, without an adequate follow-up program the supplemental fast is of only limited value. Phase two, that of maintenance, should be an essential component of treatment of this chronic disorder. Whereas the reduction phase requires a fixed caloric intake chosen for safe, rapid weight loss, the maintenance phase introduces both fixed and free calories. The focus of the behavioral and nutritional counseling continues to be the acquisition and reinforcement of skills for lifetime maintenance.

At the outset of the regimen, the physician and patient decide on a mutually acceptable and realistic ideal weight. During phase one of the therapy, the total hypocaloric intake is provided by the formula supplement. As the patient approaches her/his goal weight, s/he will begin to introduce foods to the supplement regimen. This is generally instituted after a weight loss of 50 to 75 lb. At this point the physician will calculate the total weekly caloric requirements for the individual. This figure is based on the subject's ideal weight. Of the total number of calories per week, 800 to 1,000 calories per day are designated as fixed. This number is dependent on skeleton, musculature, and occupation of the patient. In a very specific manner the patient will add food progressively to her/his diet. To the daily five portions of supplement is added one food at a designated time. The pattern changes to two foods, then three, and finally four foods. Only the specified foods may be used and only in the prescribed quantities, thus eliminating any decision-making on the part of the patient. Over a period of perhaps 4 to 5 weeks the individual will have made the transition from full supplement (5 portions) to 4 supplements plus one meal of food. If the progression is successful, behavior is controlled and weight loss continues.

Free calories are introduced to the diet at this time. As opposed to the restrictive nature of fixed calories, free calories help the patient develop a positive attitude toward food. Since there are no forbidden foods, the possibilities of cheating and guilt are eliminated. The weekly free calorie allotment is arrived at by subtracting the weekly fixed calories from the total weekly caloric requirements. The total number of free calories is divided into thirds. Initially one food of the patient's choosing is added to the diet at specific times each week. If no problems occur either with behavioral control or with weight loss, free-calorie foods are progressively added to the weekly intake until these represent one-third of the total free calories. The patient is responsible for making choices and keeping a dietary record, thus developing a sense of control over the food experience. Even with the increase in caloric load, the patient will continue to lose weight. Reduction will not be as dramatic as before, but will proceed in an acceptable manner. As the patient moves closer to achievement of her/his ideal weight, another one-third of the free calories will be added. Rarely do we introduce the final one-third of the free calories into the patient's regimen. Most often the patient has overestimated the previous two-thirds and, therefore, has already accounted for them. This can be seen in the pattern of weight loss. In the rare case that this portion is used, we incorporate it into the patient's fixed caloric intake when the four supplements are changed to food (Table 5).

In the final stages of our regimen, the use of fixed and free calories becomes dependent on the weight of the individual. A rigorous approach to maintenance is proposed. The patient should understand that for her/him weight control requires a life-time commitment. A range of weight is described for each patient. At weekly checks the free caloric allowance is defined. If the patient is in the lower range of acceptable weight, s/he is permitted the free calories. If the recorded weight is in the upper range, the free calories are withheld. Thus, the fixed calories, which are now specific foods, offer a safety valve for maintenance.

Concurrent with realimentation, the patient is taught behavior techniques that will aid her/him in the necessary change of life-style. As new behaviors are learned, they must be positively reinforced so that they become constructive habits. A patient is taught, through either individual or group therapy, to be conscious of environment, degree of·caloric intake, and emotions during eating. Traditional nutritional education and instruction in appropriate physical activity are also included in therapy sessions. Like Lindner and Blackburn (16), we have found that without the inclusion of these three elements in a modified fasting protocol, the success of the program is transient.

CONCLUSION

We believe obesity should be viewed as a chronic disease. Its treatment, like that for other chronic disorders, has problems of compliance and control. A suc-

TABLE 5. *Fixed and free calories*

Ideal weight × 10–15 × 7 = Total calories/week
− 5600 Fixed calories/week
Free calories/week
Weight gain − eliminate free calories

cessful protocol should consist of two phases: reduction and maintenance. The supplemented fast allows us a prompt and efficient way to produce weight reduction in large numbers of patients. Those patients who embark on this kind of regimen should realize that it is of little long-term value unless there are some changes in life-style. Therefore, some program of behavioral techniques must be instituted to educate patients in a modification of eating habits and physical activity. As with any chronic disorder, continual follow-up is necessary to ensure success. The frequency of this monitoring is dependent on the compliance of the patient.

The alternatives for the massively obese include continued obesity, a surgical procedure, or a combined therapy of modified fast with behavioral programming. Through our experience it seems clear that an attempt with the latter is certainly indicated. Only after this program has accumulated at least a 5-yr data base, can we be certain of its therapeutic role. To date, the results have been encouraging.

ACKNOWLEDGMENTS

The author gratefully acknowledges the contributions of Shelly Galvin and Leah Wanke in the preparation of this manuscript.

REFERENCES

1. Apfelbaum, M., Boudon, P., Lacatis, D., and Nillus, P. (1979): Effets métaboliques de la diète protidique chez 41 sujets obèses. *Presse Med.*, 78:1917–1920.
2. Blackburn, L., Bistrian, R., and Flatt, J. P. (1975): Role of a protein sparing fast in a comprehensive weight reduction programme. In: *Recent Advances in Obesity Research: 1. Proceedings of the 1st International College on Obesity. October 8–11, 1974*, edited by Alan Howard, pp. 279–281. Newman Publishing Ltd., London.
3. Bloom, W. L. (1959): Fasting as an introduction to the treatment of obesity. *Metabolism*, 8:214–220.
4. Bolinger, R. E., Lukert, B. P., Brown, R. W., Guevara, L., and Steinberg, R. (1966): Metabolic balance of obese subjects during fasting. *Arch. Intern. Med.*, 118:3–8.
5. Bray, G. A. (1977): Current status of intestinal bypass surgery in the treatment of obesity. *Diabetes*, 26:1072–1079.
6. Drenick, E. J., Swendseid, M. E., Blahd, W. H., and Tuttle, S. G. (1964): Prolonged starvation as treatment for severe obesity. *JAMA*, 187:140–145.
7. Duncan, G. G., Jenson, W. K., Cristofori, F. C., and Schless, G. L. (1963): Intermittent fasts in the correction and control of intractable obesity. *Am. J. Med. Sci.*, 245:515–520.
8. FDA (1978): Liquid protein and sudden cardiac deaths: An update. *Drug Bull.*, 8:18–19.
9. Genuth, S. (1973): Effects of oral alanine administration in fasting obese subjects. *Metabolism*, 22:927–937.
10. Genuth, S. (1979): Supplemented fasting in the treatment of obesity and diabetes. *Am. J. Clin. Nutr.*, 32:2579–2586.
11. Genuth, S., Castro, J., and Vertes, V. (1974): Weight reduction in obesity by outpatient semi-starvation. *JAMA*, 230:987–991.
12. Genuth, S., Vertes, V., and Hazelton, I. (1978): Supplemented fasting in the treatment of obesity. In: *Recent Advances in Obesity: Research 2*, edited by G. A. Bray, pp. 370–378. Newman Publishing, Ltd., London.
13. Hippocrates: *Aphorisms*. Section VII, 60. Translated in 1849 from the Greek by Francis Adams, p. 771. Sydenham Society, London, England.
14. Howard, A. A., and Baird, I. McL. (1977): A long-term evaluation of very low calorie semi-synthetic diets: An inpatient/outpatient study with egg albumin as the protein source. *Int. J. Obes.*, 1:63–78.

15. Jordan, H., and Levitz, L. (1975): A behavioral approach to the problem of obesity. *Obesity/Bariatric Med.*, 4:58–69.
16. Lindner, P. G., and Blackburn, G. L. (1976): Multidisciplinary approach to obesity utilizing fasting modified by protein sparing therapy. *Obesity/Bariatric Med.*, 5:198–215.
17. Stunkard, A., and McLaren-Hume, M. (1959): The results of treatment for obesity. *Arch. Intern. Med.*, 103:79–85.
18. Vertes, V., Genuth, S., and Hazelton, I. (1977): Supplemented fasting as a large-scale outpatient program. *JAMA*, 238:2151–2153.

Health and Obesity, edited by H. L. Conn, Jr., E. A. DeFelice, and P. Kuo. Raven Press, New York © 1983.

Drug Therapy of Obesity

Louis Lasagna

Departments of Pharmacology and Medicine, University of Rochester School of Medicine and Dentistry, Rochester, New York 14642

The use of drugs to treat obesity does not represent a particularly distinguished chapter in the history of therapeutics. Anorectic[1] drugs are scorned by many experts and poorly used by many practitioners. Why is this area of pharmacotherapy so confused and controversial?

One reason is historical. In modern times the first chemical to be marketed specifically as an antiobesity drug was dinitrophenol (DNP). DNP was not really an anorectic agent, but a chemical that was introduced because it inhibited energy-rich phosphate bond transfer and increased basal metabolic rate and oxygen consumption. Unfortunately, this agent was found to produce all kinds of toxicity, including cataracts, and was therefore withdrawn because of its potential for serious adverse effects.

A second reason is ignorance—ignorance of what true anorectic drugs can do, and what they cannot. In recent years they have been painted practically as placebos, as drugs that work both trivially and for only a short period of time. Neither assertion is correct.

In 1972 a committee was convened by the FDA to study the safety and efficacy of anorectics. This group began with some 200 double-blind controlled trials in some 10,000 subjects involved in the evaluation of 12 different drugs. The total data base, therefore, was a mishmash. The committee found that "frequently more than 50 percent of the patients dropped out of the study and were not included in the analysis." Prout, the committee chairman, has stated: "Obviously, exclusion of the dropouts led these studies to conclude greater success, since the dropout numbers largely represent treatment failures" (1).

For various reasons, therefore, this FDA group dealt with only a fraction of the data. Prout has summarized the results, based on 20 studies lasting 4 weeks, 18 studies lasting 8 weeks, and only 1 study (with 95 "starting participants") lasting 52 weeks. On average, drug-treated patients lost only 0.68 lb per week over the placebo group's loss over the first 4 weeks, 0.35 lb over the first 8 weeks, and

---

[1]This adjective will be used, although "anorexigenic" is probably more etymologically correct.

none over 52 weeks. Prout concluded that "the total impact of drug-induced weight loss over that of diet alone must be considered clinically trivial" (1).

This melange of data not only involves different drugs, but varying dosages, and no adequate consideration of such factors as initial level of obesity and dropouts. I shall later present evidence from our own group to show how faulty the committee's conclusions are in the context of specific anorectic drug use, but would like here to discuss one simple but important problem: the dropouts. Dropouts are the bane of clinical investigation, and there is no completely satisfactory way to deal with them. But on one point trial experts are agreed: you cannot ignore them. When subjects drop out because they are dissatisfied with the magnitude of therapeutic effect, there will almost invariably be more such dropouts in the placebo group. Hence to ignore them is to make the placebo look better than it deserves. This is true for anorectics, for analgesics, or for any other type of drug study where dissatisfied patients can vote with their feet. Thus a failure to count dropouts in the calculations of weight loss does not generate "greater success" for the active drug, but *less* success.

Anorectic drugs are also often written off because it is said that tolerance develops rapidly to their effects. In animals this is indeed easy to show, and complete tolerance can develop. But in patients this may or may not happen, and, if it does, increase in dosage can often overcome any loss of effect.

People have also confused decreasing rate of weight loss over time with tolerance. It is a fact that *any* weight loss program—even total starvation—will achieve more lost poundage in the early weeks than later on. But even a plateauing of effect is not necessarily a *loss* of effect. Losing weight is one thing; *keeping* it off is another. Patients who achieve a new lower, stable weight on an anorectic agent often regain at least some of this weight fairly promptly when the drug is stopped. I submit that such phenomena are not the kind of tolerance one sees in animals, where despite the continuation of anorectic drug, the treated and control groups begin after a while to have identical weights.

A third reason for the bad reputation of anorectic drugs is that some people abuse them. It is difficult to think of any central nervous system drug that is not capable of being abused by some people. There are, without question, "speed freaks" who use amphetamines or other CNS stimulants for kicks. Some of these people may show psychiatric disturbance resembling paranoid schizophrenia. But the relevant question is: how risky are oral anorectics when used properly by physicians as part of a weight control regimen? Not very, I would submit. There are, I am sorry to say, "script doctors" who prescribe stimulant anorectics for illegal purposes. In New York State, for example, where recently amphetamines have been deemed inappropriate for weight loss, 75 doctors prescribed 75% of all the amphetamines prescribed! I would wager that these doctors have now simply switched over to other drugs, some of them for improper use.

There is one troublesome syndrome, regrettably, that is occasionally seen in patients for whom amphetamines are chronically prescribed. The story is usually a stereotyped one: A young obese women is put on amphetamines. She loses weight and begins to feel like a "live person" and not a "slug" for the first time in her life. She is also able for the first time to keep up physically and socially with her peers. Over time, the dose is increased modestly but then is kept at the same level. Some years later, often because of a change in doctors, the drug is stopped, the patient balloons up in weight, becomes a "slug" again, and is terribly depressed. Going back on amphetamines is usually the only really effective treatment, but by now the patient fears that she is a drug addict and may not be willing to resume them. These patients behave as if they are suffering from an inborn deficiency of neurotransmitters similar to those released by the anorectic agent.

A final unfortunate belief is that drugs alone can manage obesity successfully. Any doctor or patient who has this belief is doomed to disappointment. Such measures as diet and exercise are ignored at one's peril.

What drugs are available for use in combatting obesity? Thyroid preparations have long been used for this purpose, in part because of the fallacious belief that obese patients are often hypometabolic. Endocrine dysfunction is not an important factor in overweight patients. Nevertheless, if one gives enough thyroid, anyone can be made to lose weight. Whether this can be accomplished with patient acceptance and safety is less clear.

The combination of thyroid preparations and modern anorectic drugs has not been adequately studied, to my knowledge, and deserves more attention from researchers in this field. There have been some perfectly dreadful combinations sold in the past, including such things as thyroid preparations, digitalis, and diuretics. These mixtures can cause serious toxicity, including death. Digitalis per se has no rationale to justify its use in the noncardiac obese. The same can be said for diuretics in the absence of fluid retention.

Bulking agents such as methylcellulose may at times reduce the intensity of feelings of hunger, but this class of drugs in general cannot be considered an important approach to effective weight loss. The same is true for human chorionic gonadotropin, which has had its advocates over the years, but in the most recent studies has appeared ineffective.

This brings us to the most widely used and most effective pharmacologic aids to weight control: the anorectic agents. I shall use this term although it is possible that these drugs may also contribute to weight control by their effects on mood and physical activity. The class name unquestionably hides considerable differences between the individual members of the class.

Fenfluramine, for example, has sedative properties not shared by the other anorectics. Furthermore, fenfluramine probably brings about its effects by a different mechanism of action than the so-called stimulant anorectics. Fenfluramine involves serotonergic systems, whereas drugs such as amphetamine, phentermine, mazindol, and diethylpropion involve the catecholamines norepinephrine and dopamine. Even within this latter group, the drugs are by no means identical.

The most popular anorectic drugs are listed in Table 1. The dosages recommended are those contained in the FDA-approved labeling. These doses tend to be on the conservative side, a fact that is made worse by the following advice in each package

TABLE 1. *Popular anorectic drugs*

Generic name	Brands	Dosage recommended on package insert
Amphetamine (racemic)	Benzedrine	5 to 30 mg daily
Dextroamphetamine	Dexedrine	5 to 30 mg daily
Amphetamine resin complex (racemic amphetamine plus dextroamphetamine)	Biphetamine	One 7.5, 12.5, or 20 mg capsule daily
Benzphetamine complex	Didrex	25 mg once a day to 50 mg t.i.d.
Chlorphentermine	Pre-Sate	65 mg (base) after first meal
Clortermine	Voranil	50 mg once a day in midmorning
Diethylpropion	Tenuate, Tepanil	25 mg t.i.d. ± one dose in midevening
Fenfluramine	Pondimin	20 mg b.i.d. to 40 mg t.i.d.
Mazindol	Sanorex	1 to 3 mg daily
Phendimetrazine	Plegine	17.5 mg b.i.d. or t.i.d. to 70 mg t.i.d.
Phenmetrazine	Preludin	50 to 75 mg b.i.d. or t.i.d.
Phentermine hydrochloride	Adipex	8 mg t.i.d. or 15 to 37.5 mg as single dose
	Fastin	30 mg as a single dose
Phentermine resin	Ionamin	15 to 30 mg daily

insert: "When tolerance to the anorectic effect develops, the recommended dose should not be exceeded in an attempt to increase the effect; rather, the drug should be discontinued." This admonition is intended to prevent drug abuse or addiction, but, if followed, it diminishes the likelihood of adequate weight loss, which sometimes requires modest increases in dose.

The package inserts for the various drugs show a strangely inconsistent approach to dosage flexibility. For instance, the labeling for phendimetrazine shows recommended dosages that range from 17.5 mg two or three times per day to 70 mg three times per day, whereas the label for clortermine says, simply: "50 mg once a day in midmorning."

There is additional irrationality in the doses for racemic amphetamine (up to 30 mg daily), dextroamphetamine, which should be twice as potent as the racemic amphetamine (also to be taken in doses up to 30 mg daily), and biphetamine, a mixture of equal amounts of dextroamphetamine and racemic amphetamine (only up to 10 mg of each daily).

The present Federal scheduling for these drugs is shown in Table 2. The FDA has in the past indicated its desire to remove obesity as an indication for the use of amphetamines.

The contraindications for the several anorectic drugs can be considered together, and include: coronary artery disease, the more severe grades of hypertension, hyperthyroidism, glaucoma, agitated states, and a history of drug abuse. As is the case with so many drugs, caution is advised in each package insert in regard to use in pregnant patients.

The adverse effects include: insomnia, dysphoria, excitement, agitation, dizziness, tremor, headache, dry mouth, unpleasant taste, impotence, hallucinations, confusion, assaultiveness, panic states, hypertension, palpitations, and tachycardia.

TABLE 2. *Present Federal scheduling for anorectic drugs*

Schedule	Drugs
II[a]	Amphetamine, dextroamphetamine, methamphetamine, phenmetrazine
III[b]	Benzphetamine, chlorphentermine, clortermine, mazindol, phendimetrazine
IV[b]	Diethylpropion, fenfluramine, phentermine

[a]II medications require a written prescription; no refills; phone prescriptions only in case of an emergency; and must be followed promptly by a signed prescription; manufacturing quotas can be imposed.

[b]III and IV medications can be ordered by phone as well as by written prescription; refills on written prescription only to a maximum of five over a period of 6 months' medication; difference between III and IV is primarily in regard to reports to DEA by manufacturer or distributor.

With fenfluramine, common side effects include drowsiness and diarrhea. Because it is a depressant, other CNS depressants, if taken concomitantly, should be used with caution.

Finally, several of the anorectics are available in delayed release or prolonged action form. Whether the convenience of such preparations compensates for the lack of flexibility in timing of dose and effect or any lack of predictability in absorption is not clear.

I should now like to describe briefly a recent trial by some of my colleagues in Rochester, since the results illustrate some important points as well as the value of an imaginative approach to the use of anorectic drugs. Weintraub had the interesting idea of combining fenfluramine and phentermine to see whether half doses of the two drugs would work as well as (or better than) full doses of each drug alone. This made sense theoretically because the side effect patterns of these drugs are different and they seem to work quite differently in animal models of obesity.

The study was a double-blind, parallel group comparison of phentermine resin (delayed release), 30 mg in the morning; fenfluramine, 20 mg three times per day; placebo; and a combination of phentermine resin, 15 mg in the morning, and fenfluramine, 30 mg before the evening meal. A double placebo technique was required because of the three dosage schedules. All participants had 3 weeks of diet only, 16 weeks of drug treatment plus diet, 4 weeks of tapering off the medication, and finally 4 weeks of follow-up off medication.

Eighty-one people with simple obesity (130 to 180% of ideal body weight) participated. Individualized diets were prescribed and instructions were repeated during the 24-week study period. Weight loss on the combination (8.4 $\pm$ 4.9 kg) was significantly greater than on placebo (4.4 $\pm$ 4.1 kg) ($p < 0.05$, Scheffé test) and equivalent to that of fenfluramine (7.5 $\pm$ 5.5 kg) or phentermine (10.0 $\pm$ 5.2 kg) alone. Percent of pretreatment weight lost was: combination, 10.1; phentermine, 11.0; fenfluramine, 8.4; and placebo, 4.9. Central nervous system and cardiovascular adverse effects were less frequent on combination than on the other active treatments. By 20 weeks (before tapering off medication) 37 participants had dropped out, 18 for reasons related to drug treatment (adverse effects, lack of efficacy, and the possibility of drug interaction). Visual analog measurements of hunger and satiety strongly favored the combination. Combining the two drugs capitalized on their pharmacodynamic differences, resulting in equivalent weight loss with fewer adverse effects and better control of appetite. The study also showed loss of weight continuing throughout 20 weeks of treatment, albeit at a slower rate as time went on. I submit that in the choice of a medication for weight control this combination should at least be considered as part of the clinical strategy.

Weintraub has followed up these patients over a period of 7 months. Of 81 participants, 32 attended the follow-up clinic and 26 responded by mail; thus 71.6% provided data. Of respondents, 84.2% gained weight after completion of the study; 21% returned to or surpassed pre-study weight. Most participants who had been on the combination or phentermine reported positive feelings about their medications; only 3 of 13 on fenfluramine and 1 of 12 on placebo did so. Participants' reasons for negative attitudes included ineffectiveness (mostly placebo patients), side effects (especially fenfluramine), and tolerance (3 each on fenfluramine and phentermine). Less than 25% of participants were continuing the diet.

There are certain principles to keep in mind when prescribing anorectic drugs.

Patients almost always do best when treated as individuals. An inflexible, stereo-typed approach to every obese patient is irrational and empirically less effective than regimens that tailor dosage and timing of dose to the individual patient on the basis of careful monitoring of response. In our experience, for example, it seems important to treat obesity as early as possible, to focus on patients who are highly motivated, and to pick different anorectic drugs depending on whether patients are anxious or depressed.

Nevertheless, attention to dosage regimen is often a more important determinant of success or failure than is the choice of drug. For instance, many obese patients are not "large breakfast" eaters, and have their big meal of the day in the evening. It is, therefore, not sensible to prescribe dosage three times daily before breakfast, lunch, and dinner. Giving the initial dose before lunch makes more sense.

Likewise, the drugs need time to be absorbed, reach the site of action, and produce an anorectic effect. An hour before the time of desired peak effect is a reasonable guess as the time to be recommended for the intake of drug, although this may differ from drug to drug and patient to patient. A range of 30 to 90 min before desired peak effect probably encompasses the needs of most patients.

Since most of the available drugs are central nervous system stimulants, having the patient take the drug late in the day will often interfere with sleep. The time of the evening meal and of bedtime may be modified to advantage, as well as the timing and amount of the last dose. If these maneuvers fail, a hypnotic can also be used.

The stimulant effects of anorectics are not entirely deleterious. The initiation and maintenance of a weight control program can be a depressing experience for many obese patients, and the mild emotional lift provided by many anorectic drugs helps some patients through a difficult situation. The price paid for the benefit is that a few patients will abuse the drugs to achieve euphoria.

A short-term approach to the control of obesity makes no more sense when drugs are used than when they are not. Most obese people have less trouble losing weight than in keeping the lost weight off. Hence, each physician must decide for himself what role he envisages for anorectic drugs in his long-term approach. He can, for instance, turn to anorectic drugs only if nondrug regimens fail, or after the effects of dietary restriction have plateaued. Or he may wish to use an anorectic at the initiation of a weight control regimen, to help get the patient off to a good start, and then stop the drug. Or he may decide to use anorectic drugs very briefly in patients who have little response to them, or who cannot obtain therapeutic benefit without intolerable side effects, but continue drug use in patients who experience benefit without serious untoward effects. For most chronic diseases, effective drugs are taken for long periods of time. Obesity is a chronic disease.

Reinforcement is important in this area of human activity, as in all others. One of the reasons for the success of such programs as Weight Watchers and Diet Workshop is the need for their clients to be checked repeatedly and regularly on their progress. The same is true for physician-based programs, which means that long periods between visits and a reliance on telephone prescription renewals are not likely to lead to success.

REFERENCE

1. Prout, T. E. (1980): The myth of the usefulness of amphetamines in the long-term management of obesity. In: *Controversies in Therapeutics*, edited by L. Lasagna, pp. 184–190. W. B. Saunders Co., Philadelphia.

Health and Obesity, edited by H. L. Conn, Jr.,
E. A. DeFelice, and P. Kuo. Raven Press,
New York © 1983.

Surgical Treatment of Obesity

George L. Blackburn and *Marijean M. Miller

*Department of Surgery, Harvard Medical School and *Nutrition Support Service, Cancer
Research Institute, New England Deaconess Hospital, Boston, Massachusetts 02215*

The surgical treatment of obesity has evolved over the past 20 years into an effective management technique for the morbidly obese. Three basic procedures will be examined: the jejunoileal bypass, the gastric bypass, and gastroplasty. These operative solutions are reserved for the treatment of those "morbidly" obese patients who are >200% of their ideal weight. Our preferred procedure is the gastric bypass using a Roux-en-y gastrojejunostomy, 30-cc pouch, and a 1.2-cm anastamosis. This procedure has emerged as an effective treatment for the morbidly obese causing weight loss (34 to 100% of initial excess, mean = 46 kg), an increased lean body mass/body weight ratio from the first postsurgical month, and minimized complications. The success of surgical intervention is dependent on a multidisciplinary approach. Surgery is best utilized as an adjunct to a comprehensive treatment program stressing improvement of lifestyle through control of calorie intake, behavior modification, and increased physical activity.

OBESITY: MORBIDITY AND MORTALITY RATES

Obesity is a disease predisposing the patient to a wide variety of chronic illnesses (Table 1). Three million men and 4.5 million women in the United States are significantly obese with weights 30 to 40% above the ideal. These people have a 40% increased risk of mortality (30,54). The relation between excess weight and mortality risk is even more dramatic in those considered "morbidly" obese, as defined by weights >200% of ideal. Morbid obesity predisposes patients to a 12-fold increase in mortality risk (19).

Diabetes mellitus and hypertension are the two most common of the chronic illnesses associated with severe obesity. Eighty percent of adult-onset diabetics (12

TABLE 1. *Conditions associated with morbid obesity*

Diabetes mellitus	Degenerative arthritis
Hypertension	Gallbladder disease
Coronary heart disease	Infertility
Congestive heart disease	Hyperlipoproteinemia
Restrictive lung disease	Psychosocial incapacity

million Americans) are obese. A weight 45% in excess of ideal constitutes a 30-fold increase in risk for diabetes mellitus (55). The Framingham Study revealed a similar relation between excess weight and hypertension (27). For each 10% increment in body weight, there is a 6.5 mm increase in systolic blood pressure, a 12 mg/dl increase in plasma cholesterol, and a 2 mg/dl rise in fasting blood sugar (6). In a study of 200 morbidly obese men, Drenick noted that the majority of deaths were from the life-debilitating conditions associated with obesity. He emphasized that "the obese state caused the commonly occurring degenerative disease to begin at an earlier age, to progress more rapidly, and to become life-threatening more frequently" (19).

THE JUSTIFICATION FOR SURGICAL TREATMENT

Medical weight loss programs emphasizing a multidisciplinary approach can be successful in reducing the mortality risk of the moderately obese patient through weight reduction. However, for the morbidly obese patient, even the best of the medical weight loss and maintenance programs reported in the literature cannot sustain the magnitude of weight loss necessary for treatment. Surgical treatment for the disease of morbid obesity was developed as an adjunct to dietary therapy.

In 1959 Stunkard and McLaren-Hume (53) initiated the evaluation of medical weight loss programs in their classic paper reporting the limited success of balanced deficit dieting in the treatment of obesity. In 25% of the outpatients studied a short-term weight loss of 9.1 kg occurred. In only 5% of the patients the weight loss exceeded 18.2 kg (53).

Follow-up studies show that even when weight loss was achieved, long-term maintenance of weight loss was generally poor. Only 5% retained their weight loss after several years (54). These data are consistent with the common observation that most severely obese people have attempted a variety of medical weight loss techniques with little success.

Recent papers evaluating an integrated approach combining behavior modification and modified fasting have reported more promising weight loss and maintenance results. In a 4.5-year follow-up study, Bistrian and Sherman (5) reported one-third of their patients maintained a weight loss of 18.2 kg. A multidisciplinary approach to obesity therapy stressing modification of food habits, physical activity, and reduced calorie intake has been proven superior to diet therapy alone (25,31). The best weight loss and maintenance results reported in the literature have been with the multidisciplinary approach utilized at the Center for Nutritional Research located in Boston. This group reported a significant weight loss of 40 lb in 52% of 338 patients studied over a period of 5 to 7 years (39).

Medical dietary regimes can be of significant value to the patient who is moderately obese. A successful loss of 40 lb will produce a marked reduction in the mortality risk of these patients. Dieting in the moderately obese can thus bring patients within 130% of ideal weight. However, even the maximized effort of such medical dietary regimes fall far short of the treatment requirements of the morbidly obese person who needs to lose >100 lb.

The effectiveness of each surgical procedure can be examined in terms of the magnitude of weight loss produced and the associated complications. In addition, the quality of weight loss (fat mass versus lean body mass) as assessed by K^{40} and T_2O body composition studies can also be determined (20,47).

Successful surgical management is expected to produce a quality (predominantly fat) 10 to 15 lb/month weight loss in a period of 9 to 15 months (7). An effective surgical procedure combined with a comprehensive obesity therapy including nutritional education, diet counseling, exercise planning, and behavior modification (3,25) will produce the best results.

Candidates for surgical treatment will meet at least one of the following criteria: (a) weight at least 300 lb, (b) weight 100 lb in excess of ideal, and (c) or weight >200% of ideal as determined by the standard weight/height charts (15). Patients must also demonstrate an inability to succeed at weight loss with dietary control, a stable adult life pattern, and be between the age of 18 and 50 years. In addition, the patient should have an absence of serious heart disease, inflammatory bowel disease, and hepatic or renal dysfunction.

AN OVERVIEW OF THE OBJECTIVES OF THE JEJUNOILEAL AND GASTRIC BYPASS OPERATIONS

The jejunoileal bypass, gastric bypass, and gastroplasty operations are designed to induce weight loss by very different means. Evolved from the extinct jejunocolic bypass, the *jejunoileal bypass* is designed to shorten the intestinal tract and, by reducing intestinal absorptive capacity, to induce weight loss despite intake at presurgery levels (42, Fig. 1). The intention of the *gastric bypass* and *gastroplasty* operations is to restrict food intake by reducing stomach size (35, Fig. 2). The absorptive properties of the intestine are not modified by the gastric bypass, rather the stomach size is reduced to restrict intake. In the gastric bypass, food passes into a limb of jejunum, thus excess carbohydrates, particularly sugar, produce the

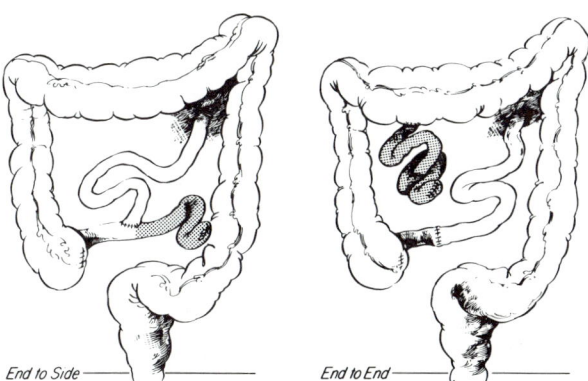

End to Side   End to End

FIG. 1. **Left:** Jejunoileal bypass: end-to-side. **Right:** Jejunoileal bypass: end-to-end. (From Maini, ref. 33, with permission.)

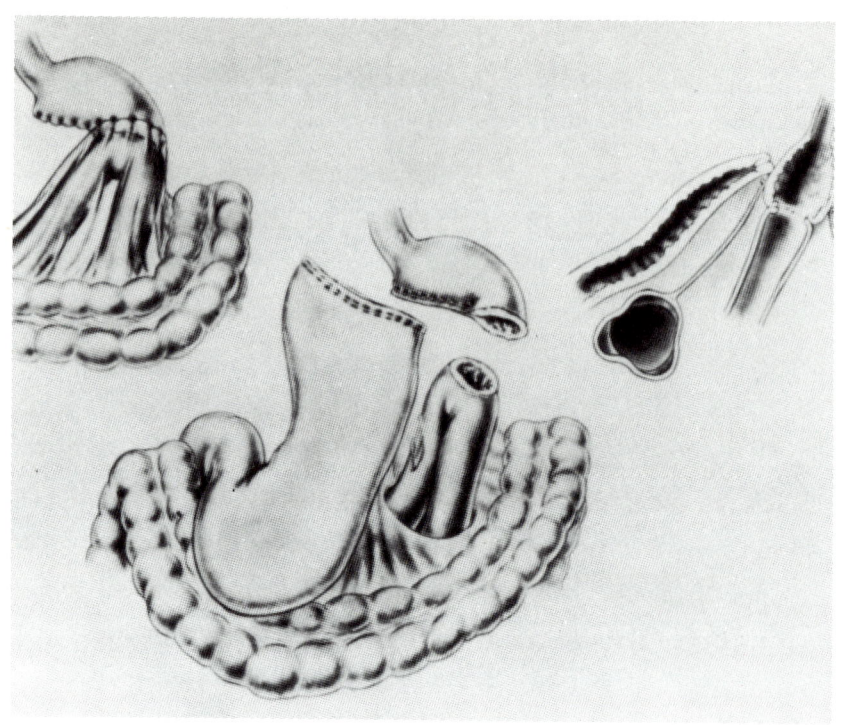

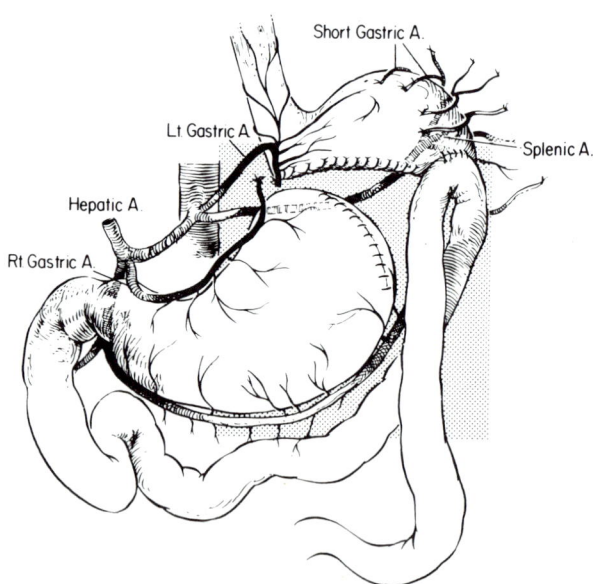

Short Gastric A.

Lt Gastric A.

Splenic A.

Hepatic A.

Rt Gastric A.

FIG. 2. Top: The gastric bypass: early version with transected stomach. (From Mason and Ito, ref. 35a, with permission.) **Bottom:** The gastric bypass: detail of arterial access. (From Maini, ref. 34, with permission.)

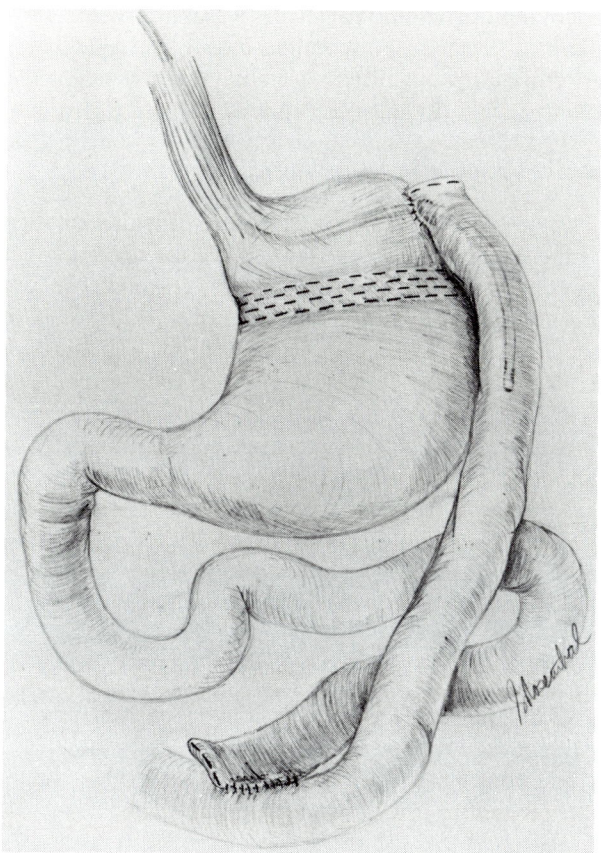

FIG. 2. continued. The gastric bypass: present version with stapling procedure (the stomach is not transected). (From Bothe et al., ref. 7, with permission.)

dumping syndrome (16), which rapidly conditions a change in dietary habits in the patient conducive to sustained weight loss. In contrast, the gastroplasty is merely a partial partitioning of the stomach (30- to 50-cc pouch) with a 1.2-cm outlet into the lower stomach. Thus, with gastroplasty, food intake is controlled by pouch and outlet size without the benefit of the feedback conditioning of the dumping syndrome.

THE HISTORY, COMPLICATIONS, AND CLINICAL UTILITY OF THE SURGICAL PROCEDURES

Jejunocolic Bypass

Payne et al. were the first to perform the jejunoileal shunt as a surgical technique to produce weight reduction (43). Intolerable metabolic complications soon led to the abandonment of this operation. Weight loss was impressive, but was complicated by intractable diarrhea, abdominal discomfort, electrolyte depletion, and liver failure (42). The severity of electrolyte disturbances required operation reversal in a substantial number of patients. In some, death was reported due to liver failure.

Jejunoileal Bypass

Payne and DeWind published the first report of the jejunoileal bypass as a modification of the jejunocolic bypass (42). Since the operation's initial development, several groups have performed the bypass, changing the orientation of the jejunum to ileum anastomosis (see Fig. 1), from *end-to-side* to *end-to-end*, and the lengths of the jejunum and the ileum segments used. The *end-to-end jejunoileal bypass* is generally performed at present with the lengths of jejunum and ileum utilized varying from 12 to 15 inches and from 4 to 8 inches, respectively (47,48). Several groups have reported better results with the end-to-end jejunoileal bypass than with the end-to-side bypass (9,11,49), despite the fact that both procedures are associated with severe complications (8). Body composition studies suggest that the use of the 12 inch jejunum and 6 to 8 inch ileum length minimizes the lean body mass weight loss associated with this operation (49), which may be as great as 50% of the total body weight lost in the first 6 months (9).

End-to-Side Bypass

The 1969 paper of Payne and DeWind described their experience with 58 patients undergoing the end-to-side bypass. Fourteen inches of the jejunum were anastomised to 4 inches of the terminal ileum (Fig. 1, left). Twelve other patients received the bypass procedures with longer lengths of jejunum and ileum, but the 14 to 4 shunt produced the best weight loss (42).

In a more recent study the authors reported their experience with an additional 82 patients, using the same jejunoileal bypass (44). Weight loss was satisfactory but was generally associated with hypokalemia, diarrhea, anal pain with hemorrhoids, ease of fatigue, thirst, and nausea. Sequential liver biopsies tended to reveal an increase in fat in the early postoperative period. Renal calculi, acute cholecystitis with cholelithiasis, and polyarthritis were also noted. The overall mortality rate was reported to be 6%.

The end-to-side bypass procedure is as follows: exposure is best obtained through a large transverse supraumbilical incision, with division of the rectus muscles. Liver biopsy is carried out routinely after exploration of the abdominal cavity. The ligament of Trietz is identified and the jejunum is carefully measured along the mesenteric border and divided at the desired point. The distal end of the bypass jejunum is closed in two layers and fixed to the mesentery to avoid intussusception. The end of the proximal jejunum is anastomosed to the side of the ileum, 4 inches from the ileocecal valve.

A clinical and metabolic appraisal of the end-to-side jejunoileal bypass on 11 patients reported good clinical results in only 7 out of 11 patients. Specific nutritional deficits and fatty livers were observed in some patients and were of concern to the authors (49). Subsequent work by Scott et al. in 1975 found the end-to-side jejunoileal bypass to be inferior to the end-to-end jejunoileal bypass because it produced a more gradual weight loss (47). This weight loss plateaued after 12 to 18 months at levels above the ideal range.

End-to-End Bypass

In 1965 Sherman et al. proposed modifying the end-to-side bypass because he suspected some of the undesirable side effects (weight gain, bacterial overgrowth in the bypassed segment, etc.) resulted from reflux of intestinal contents into the excluded intestine. The revision devised was an end-to-end jejunoilostomy with an ileocecostomy to allow for drainage of the defunctionalized intestinal loop (46,50, see Fig. 1, right). Brill et al. utilized a 12 inch jejunum to 6 inch ileum end-to-end bypass in 14 patients. When these results were compared to 11 patients given the 14 to 4 Payne and DeWind procedure, a larger percentage of those with end-to-end bypass had a satisfactory weight loss of 20 to 40% (13/14 versus 5/11) (9).

Various lengths of jejunum and ileum have been utilized in the end-to-end bypass operations performed by different groups. Buchwald et al. performed an end-to-end anastomosis between 40 cm (15 inches) of jejunum and 4 cm (1.6 inches) of ileum with the bypassed segment draining into the cecum (11). Benfield et al. anastomosed 40 cm of jejunum to 10 cm of terminal ileum allowing for drainage of the bypassed segment into the transverse colon (4). The 1975 Scott et al. study previously mentioned specifically compared procedures in which various lengths of jejunum were anastomised to ileum in end-to-end bypass operations (47). Three end-to-end procedures (12 to 12 inch, 12 to 6 inch, 12 to 8 inch) were compared to the Payne and DeWind 14 to 4 inch end-to-side procedure. Eighty-one percent of the 12 to 8 inch group, and 60% of the 12 to 6 inch group had "good" results, although all groups except the 12 to 8 inch group had depressed lean body mass to weight ratios from presurgery values until the sixth postsurgical month.

Complications

Bray presented an excellent review of the surgical complications associated with the jejunoileal bypass (8). A summary is depicted in Table 2. Complications affected 40% of the patients. The shorter the intestine the greater the weight loss and the number of nutritional complications.

Operative mortality has been attributed to liver failure, pulmonary embolism, cardiac failure, pancreatitis, hypocalcemia, sepsis, and wound dehiscence. At present, only a team of physicians, psychologists, and surgeons working within the guidelines of clinical investigation should carry out this procedure. Adequate preoperative evaluation is imperative and postoperatively the high frequency of complications will require long-term monitoring.

The leading cause of death in jejunoileal bypass patients is liver failure. The obese are predisposed to fatty livers and this condition is aggravated by the jeju-

TABLE 2. *Complications of jejunoileo bypass*

Complications	Percent
Early	
Operative mortality	0–6.5
Pulmonary emboli	1–6
Wound infection	2–10
Gastrointestinal hemorrhage	0–6
Renal failure	0–9
Later	
Urinary calculi	3–30
Liver disease	0–14
Anemia	0–3
Acute cholecystitis	0–7
Intestinal obstruction	0–3.5
Minor	
Diarrhea	100
Minor electrolyte abnormalities	40–80
Hypoproteinemia	40–100
Vomiting	10–80
Polyarthritis	0–6
Hair loss	0–100

From Bray et al. (ref. 8), with permission.

noileal bypass (18). Generally, 50% of obese patients have liver histology, but in the morbidly obese a fatty liver is observed in 75% of all cases (11,42,56). Liver disease is a long-term complication of the jejunoileal bypass, affecting as many as 14% of patients (8,10). Since liver disease requires some time to develop, long-term preventative postoperative follow-up must be conducted.

As Maini (33) described, the earliest manifestation of liver disease is an alteration of enzyme function, hepatomegaly, and hypoalbuminemia. Serum bilirubin will rise with progressive liver failure. In severe cases, cirrhosis, hepatic coma, ascites, and death may occur. These changes can be detected most reliably by early liver scan and biopsy. Liver biopsies at 6-month intervals are strongly recommended until weight loss has stabilized for 1 year and hepatic morphology has been demonstrated as normal or stable. Although the etiology remains unclear, hepatic steatosis may be related to (a) protein deficiency, (b) absorption of toxic bile acids (lithocholic acid and chenodeoxycholic acid), (c) absorption of bacterial toxins, (d) insult by alcohol ingestion (past or present), and (e) the length of the bypassed segment (33).

Dietary treatment of liver failure

In the early stages hepatic dysfunction can be treated by increasing oral protein intake. With more severe hepatic dysfunction, hospitalization and intravenous hyperalimentation are indicated. In some cases restoration of intestinal continuity is required to ensure survival. Heimburger et al. proposed treating hepatic steatosis by administering glucose-free amino acids (26). This encourages mobilization of fat, while protein loss is minimized (2). Liver failure most frequently occurs in the first postsurgical year. One to 3% of all jejunoileal bypass patients have liver failure.

Avoidance of pulmonary embolus

Pulmonary embolus is the second most common complication. Elevations in serum fatty acid levels have been implicated in the genesis of the hypercoagulable state and in pulmonary emboli (8). Serum fatty acid levels should be monitored. Mason et al. have stressed that bypass patients should not be fasted immediately prior to surgery because fasting elevates the concentration of serum fatty acids (36). Monitoring of AT III levels appears to be a sensitive index for identification of patients with a high risk for thrombosis.

Morbidity

Impaired absorptive capacity and rapid transit time are the two major factors causing electrolyte imbalances after the jejunoileal bypass. Eight to 20 liquid bowel movements per day may be experienced by the patient when eating is resumed postoperatively. The liquid bowel movements gradually decrease to 4 to 10 semi-formed stools per day. Hypoglycemia, hypokalemia, hypermagnesemia, dehydration, and acidosis may be observed in association with hypoproteinemia and anemia. As these complications can be life-threatening, meticulous biochemical monitoring, including records of stool and urine losses, is required.

As a preventative measure, patients should receive oral supplements of calcium and potassium as well as antidiarrheal agent at discharge. Bray et al. noted that some patients have difficulty maintaining normal serum concentrations of potassium and calcium as long as 2 to 3 years after their operations (8). Potassium is best provided by K-lyte, an effervescent liquid. Calcium can be supplied with Tums® or Titralac®. In the postoperative period, foods high in potassium are recommended (Table 3). As the frequency of diarrhea and electrolyte abnormalities decrease, these supplements can be reduced.

Shizgal et al. have recently reported that 25% of 44 patients who received a 15 to 5 inch end-to-side bypass developed body compositions characteristic of protein malnutrition with contracted mass and an expanded extracellular mass (51). The authors determined by multiple isotope dilution techniques that in the 11 who were

TABLE 3. *High potassium content foods*

Cantaloupe	Artichoke	Potatoes, sweet
Cherries, raw	Asparagus, frozen	Potatoes, white
Grapes, raw	Broccoli, fresh	Radishes
Nectarines	Brussel sprouts	Soybeans
Oranges	Carrots, raw	Squash, winter
Peaches, raw/dried	Cowpeas, cooked	Apricots, canned/dried
Strawberries, fresh	Dried split peas	Avocado
Juices	Parsnips	Blackberries, raw
Pumpkin		Bananas

protein malnourished, weight loss consisted significantly of both body fat and mass. Whereas body weight decreased 27%, body cell mass had decreased 22%. This study explains the need for a postbypass diet containing adequate protein.

Impairment of fat absorption has been determined consistently in several operative series (4,49). Fat excretion can be correlated with the length of the residual jejunum in continuity.

Late complications

In addition to liver disease, urinary calculi are found in 3 to 30% of postbypass patients. These calculi are almost always composed of calcium oxalate, and, thus, patients should probably avoid foods high in oxalate content (Table 4).

Polyarthritis and polyarthralgia occur in approximately 10% of all patients and is more frequently seen 3 to 6 months after surgery. The symptoms, if severe, will usually subside with small doses of corticosteroids.

"Bypass enteritis," as described by Passaro et al., can occur 2 to 6 weeks after the bypass and is characterized by severe abdominal pain, diarrhea, and a tender abdomen (41). On radiologic examination, distended bowel loops and/or free air in the peritoneal cavity are observed. The syndrome responds well to intravenous antibiotics and, for this reason, is believed to be related to an overgrowth of enteric flora, particularly anaerobes.

Weight Loss After Jejunoileal Bypass

In the first year postoperatively, the minimum weight loss reported has ranged between 30 and 150 lb (4,17). Weight loss decreases the second year and, thereafter, begins to stabilize. Benfield et al. observed a greater weight loss in patients with an end-to-end bypass, although differences were not significant (4). Body composition studies after surgery show that as great as 25% of lean body mass is lost in the first 6 months. This may represent 50% of the total body weight lost (9,47). Such a significant reduction in lean body mass is not desirable.

In summary, a "good" result of 100-lb weight loss without rehospitalization or reoperation exists in 35% of patients when the jejunoileal bypass is performed by a medical center team that diligently continues follow-up monitoring of diet com-

TABLE 4. *High oxalate content foods*

Currants	Beans
Concord grapes	Beets
Gooseberries	Spinach
Raspberries	Chard
Figs	Endive
Plums	Okra
Rhubarb	Cocoa
Tomatoes	Tea
Beet greens	Almonds
Chocolate	Cashews

pliance and biochemical status. Since complications remain substantial in 25% of the patients and are considerably greater than those observed with the gastric bypass procedure, the use of the jejunoileal bypass is diminishing.

Gastric Bypass

Mason and Ito proposed the gastric bypass operation as an intake reducing surgical treatment for the morbidly obese (35). The operation is a modification of the Billroth II gastrectomy originally introduced in 1884 as a surgical treatment for acid peptic disease, in which stomach resection for ulceration was discovered to result in a side effect of intake deficiency (37).

In the original gastric bypass operation, the stomach was actually transected (Fig. 2a). Alden (1) introduced a stapling division procedure whereby transection of the stomach and the major risk of interfering with the blood supply at the anastomotic site could be avoided (Fig. 2b,2c). The stapling procedure allowed for reduced operating time and, thus, minimized operative complications. The gastric bypass operation preferred by our group is a Roux-en-y gastrojejunostomy (23).

The current gastroplasty operation, a modification of the gastric bypass, is most successfully applied by Gomez (21, 22). Four rows of staples are inserted with a double application of the TA-90 stapler (#4.5 staples). The operative procedure creates a 60-cc fundic reservoir with a 12-mm channel located on the greater curvature of the stomach (Fig. 3). Gastroplasty is simply a partitioning of the stomach and, thus, does not produce the "dumping syndrome" beneficial to weight control in those with the gastric bypass. Precise details of the gastroplasty operative procedure using the seromuscular suture support technique are reported by Gomez (21). Currently, outlets are created on the lesser curve (37), middle (32), and greater curves (22). Concern exists as to whether staple line disruption and dilation of outlet can be prevented.

The Gastric Bypass Within an Integrated Treatment Program

The gastric bypass operation is a preferred surgical treatment for morbid obesity. Bothe et al. (7) has presented a detailed account of the operative care utilized at the New England Deaconess Hospital within a comprehensive, multidisciplinary obesity treatment program. Patients undergoing the gastric bypass experience a significant change in eating behavior as a result of this operation. It is imperative, therefore, that patients receive adequate preoperative evaluation and surveillance after surgery. Adequate behavior/personality assessment, laboratory evaluation, and a thorough physical examination are essential (Table 5).

In brief, the gastric bypass procedure is as follows: After induction of general anesthesia, additional monitoring devices are applied. A urinary catheter is inserted and a central venous and arterial catheter are placed. The skin is incised in the midline, the subcutaneous fat is separated bluntly, and the peritoneum is entered. The abdomen is completely explored. A special self-retaining circular retraction system is used (Buckwalter-Retractor). A TA-90 stapler is placed such that a small

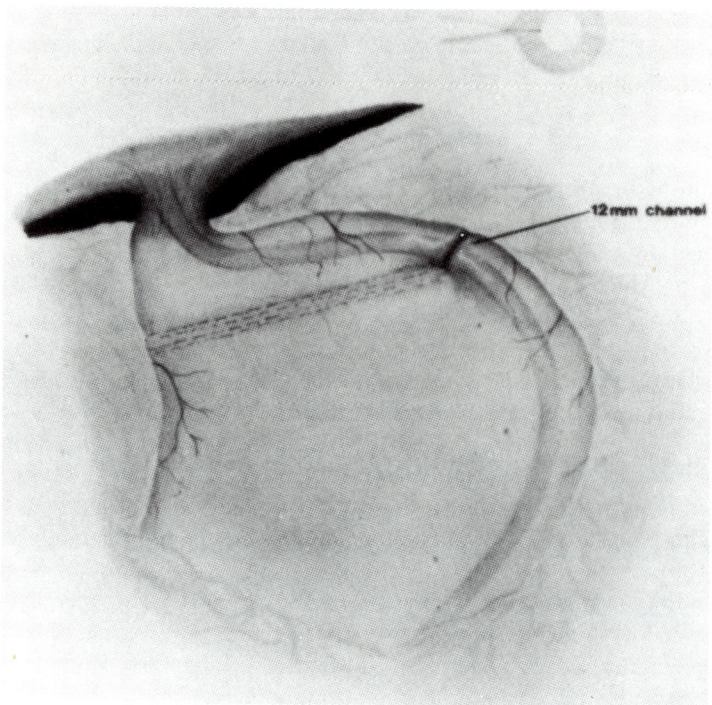

12 mm channel

FIG. 3. Gastroplasty. (From Gomez, ref. 21, with permission.)

gastric pouch less than 30 cc is created by direct measurement (1). Two double rows of staples are applied. The stomach is not divided. At a suitable distance from the ligament of Trietz, the small bowel is divided, and a standard Roux-en-y limb is formed. This procedure can be facilitated by the use of an anastomotic stapler. The limb is led on an atecolic or retrocolic fashion to the region of the gastric pouch and is anastomosed to the lateral portion of the gastric pouch on the greater curve just above the staple line. The retrocolic route is more usual due to fat content in the abdomen. The completed operation is shown in Fig. 2c (7,34).

A summary of postoperative procedures is shown in Table 6. High suspicion of an anastomotic leak or subphrenic abscess should exist if the patient produces no urinary ketones, blood sugar is > 110 mg, and, in particular, if a pulse rate ≥120 exists. The presence of fever, tachycardia, and tachypnia must be evaluated carefully. If these symptoms suggest an anastomotic leak, an immediate gastrographic swallow is performed to differentiate a fistula from atelectasis.

Our follow-up care is in complete agreement with the NIH Consensus Conference (54) on long-term care for gastric bypass patients. To receive the long-term results desired from this operation, patient compliance to the new diet, behavior modification efforts, and exercise program are crucial.

TABLE 5. *Preoperative care*

The following studies are completed or data collected:
Office
  HELP Medical History and Physical Status Form
  Obesity Questionnaire: Short and Long (Lindner) Forms
  Minesota Multiphasic Personality Inventory/Profile of Mood Status/Stress Index
  Astrand Exercise Bicycle Test
Hospital
  Inpatient or admission laboratory tests including:
    Chem 20, CBC with differential, urinalysis, platelet count, PT, PTT, AT_{III} B-12,
    folate, iron, TIBC, CVS, and HDL cholesterol
  Electrocardiogram
  Outpatient chest X-ray, upper-GI series, double-dose oral cholecystogram,
    and pulmonary function tests: Short form with room air arterial blood gases
Mini-dose heparin: 5,000 units every 12 hr
Bowel preparation: One bottle magesium citrate the day prior to surgery, Fleet's enema
    the evening before surgery.
Intravenous catheter, preferably central (subclavian or internal jugular) with normal saline.
Start intravenous evening prior to surgery if early case, or early morning if afternoon
    case
Cefazolin, 1 g with preoperative medications

Adapted from Bothe et al. ref. 7, with permission.

TABLE 6. *Postoperative care*

Intravenous infusions: Maintain carbohydrate-free regimen (no dextrose).
No patient should be extubated until in the recovery room.
Nasogastric tube to low suction with gentle (10 cc saline) every 6 hr.
Irrigate catheter jejunostomy with 10 cc saline every 6 hr.
Urine from Foley-sugar and acetone, specific gravity every 8 hr.
Remove Foley as soon as practical.
Keep accurate intake and output records, and weigh patient at least every other day.
Continue mini-heparin dose as preoperatively.
Continue antibiotic for two additional doses only.
Ensure that chest X-ray film confirms the position of the central catheter.
Use nasotracheal suction as needed with low threshold for fever or pulmonary changes.
Schedule upper-GI series before discharge. Requisition must ask radiologist to measure
    volume of pouch.

From Bothe et al. ref. 7, with permission.

Complications with the Gastric Bypass and Gastroplasty

Buckwalter examined the complications associated with the gastric bypass operation (13, 14). Although 18% developed postoperative complications, he concluded these were "few and trivial" when compared to the complications associated with the jejunoileal bypass. Complications included anastomotic leak, atelectasis, transient gastrojejunostomy obstruction, and intraabdominal abscess. The problems of wound infection, dehiscence, and pulmonary embolism were comparable to those described for the jejunoileal bypass.

The most serious complication is an anastomotic leak. Anastomotic leak can occur because of compromised circulation to the gastric pouch. If the left gastric artery is tied close to its origin from the celiac axis, ischemia of the fundic segment results because the short gastric vessels have also been occluded (34). When the left gastric artery is divided just distal to the takeoff of the ascending esophageal artery, the latter may be the only blood vessel supplying the gastric pouch. Edema in the Hoffmeister pouch may further contribute to ischemia. A careful division of the short gastric pouch and manual preparation of the anastomosis are important. Leaving a stump catheter under the left diaphragm near the anastomosis in high-risk patients may avoid the need for reoperation.

Vomiting is frequent in gastric bypass patients, but usually is secondary to eating too much, too rapidly. Behavior modification within an integrated treatment program will avoid this problem, which can, in severe instances, lead to electrolyte disturbances. When vomiting is secondary to stomal dysfunction, it is usually treated by short-term nasogastric suction and intravenous fluids.

As a late complication, 1.8% of patients develop stomal ulceration after gastric bypass using a loop gastrojejunostomy (38). Anemia is an early indication of stomal ulcer that suggests the need for investigation by endoscopy. In cases where medical therapy is unsuccessful, vagotomy is necessary. The incidence of stomach ulceration is low because a small fundic pouch necessarily has fewer parietal cells and, thereby, less acid secretion. In addition, Mason and Ito (35) have shown that the constant flow of acid from the excluded gastric segment into the duodenum maintains acid secretion at a low level by inhibiting gastrin release.

Complications with gastroplasty are found in approximately 20% of patients and include: wound sepsis, dehiscence, acute perforation of the pouch, subphrenic abscess, pneumonia, and atelectasis (21). Late complications, over a period of 1 year, occurred in 16% of patients and consisted primarily of revisions (4.5%) because of staple-line disruption, broken suture, stenosis of the channel or rehospitalization for vomiting. The gastroplasty remains to be established as a definitive procedure for the surgical treatment of morbid obesity due to the high frequency of staple disruption, dilation of the outlet, and the limited long-term (2 to 5 year) weight loss.

Weight Loss with Gastroplasty and Gastric Bypass

After gastroplasty using the seromuscular suture support technique, patients experienced a 40-kg weight loss, which reduced their excess weight to approximately 140% of ideal (21). Although Gomez reports good results with gastroplasty, others have been less successful. A recent study has also found limited success in four modifications of gastroplasty (32). The one procedure that was acceptable produced "good" results in only 44% of patients. Two of these procedures were completely unacceptable, producing unsatisfactory weight loss. Of those with unsatisfactory results, 16% had obstruction of the stoma requiring intake through the enterostomy tube for longer than 1 month. MacLean concluded that although the principle of limiting oral intake is attractive and avoids the malnutrition and liver failure associated with the jejunoileal bypass, no reliable method yet exists in the gastroplasty procedure for ensuring the permanent, small stoma essential for prolonged weight loss. Laws and Piantadosi reported better weight loss with the gastric bypass than with gastroplasty (28). More recently, Lechner and Callender conducted a prospective randomized comparison of the gastric bypass and gastroplasty operations in 100 patients (29). The authors reported weight loss with the gastric bypass to be 35% greater.

The gastric bypass series by Mason reports an average weight loss over a 3-year period of approximately 36 kg. One-third of the patients will have lost 50 kg by the end of 3 years (38). Palombo et al. (40) reported an average 46-kg weight loss 12 months after gastric bypass surgery. Palombo also studied weight loss composition in this group of patients. Lean body mass was estimated from K^{40} measurements and urine creatinine during weight loss for a period of 1.5 years. The weight loss phase lasted approximately 1 year during which time 34% of the initial weight was lost. Lean body mass was found to account for 32% of the total weight loss at 1 month, 11% at 6 months, and only 3% at 1 year. Overall lean body mass as percent of total body weight increased from 35% presurgery to 51% 1.5 years postsurgery. Actual lean body mass content increased steadily from the first postsurgical month. These weight loss composition findings are in direct contrast to those associated with the jejunoileal bypass (52). Lean body mass losses represented from 30 to 55% of the total body weight lost after 6 months in the two most successful jejunoileal bypass groups (III and IV) studied by Scott et al. (47).

Evaluation of the Jejunoileal Bypass and Gastric Bypass

Comparative studies of the gastric bypass and jejunoileal bypass were conducted (1, 12, 24, 45) with the authors expressing a preference for the gastric bypass procedure. Buckwalter went as far as to state that the "jejunoileal bypass is no longer an acceptable or defensible operation because of the prohibitive morbidity" associated with the operation. Alden compared 100 of 14- to 4-inch jejunoileal bypass patients with 100 gastric bypass patients in which 90% of the stomach was bypassed and reported that the long-term complications of the jejunoileal bypass were of greater frequency, duration, and seriousness. Whereas jejunoileal patients generally lost 31% of initial weight and had a 32% rehospitalization rate, gastric bypass patients lost 36% of their initial weight and had only a 12% rehospitalization rate. In the gastric bypass group, there was a low incidence of peptic ulcer (1.6%), dumping syndrome, and vomiting, but the severe complications of the jejunoileal bypass—liver disease, rectal problems, urinary calculi, etc.—were absent.

CONCLUSION

The surgical treatment of the morbidly obese has been developed over a period of approximately 20 years. The three basic procedures the jejunoileal bypass, gastric bypass, and gastroplasty have been designed to aid those unable to benefit from multidisciplinary diet therapy alone. The gastric bypass operation must be considered the most satisfactory procedure to date, because of its effectiveness in producing quality weight loss without severe complications.

REFERENCES

1. Alden, J. F. (1977): Gastric and jejunoileal bypass. *Arch. Surg.*, 112:799–806.
2. Blackburn, G. L., Flatt, J. P., and Hensle, T. W. (1976): Peripheral amino acid infusions. In: *Total Parenteral Nutrition*, edited by J. Fischer, pp. 363–394. Little, Brown & Co., Boston.
3. Blackburn, G. L., and Greenberg, I. (1978): Multidisciplinary approach to adult obesity therapy. *Int. J. Obes.*, 2:133–142.
4. Benfield, J. R., Greenway, F. L., Bray, G. A., Barry, R. E., Lechago, J., Mena, J., and Schedewie, H. (1976): Experience with jejunoileal bypass for obesity. *Surg. Gynecol. Obstet.*, 143:401–410.
5. Bistrian, B. R., and Sherman, M. (1978): Results of the treatment of obesity with a protein-sparing modified fast. *Int. J. Obes.*, 2:143–148.
6. Bjerkedahl, T. (1957): Overweight and hypertension. *Acta Med. Scand.*, 159:13–26.
7. Bothe, A., Bistrian, B. R., Greenberg, I., and Blackburn, G. L. (1979): Energy regulation in morbid obesity by multidisciplinary therapy. *Surg. Clin. North Am.*, 59:1017–1031.
8. Bray, G. A., Barry, R. E., Benfield, J. R., Castelnuovo-Tedesco, P., Drenick, E. J., and Passaro, E. (1976): Intestinal bypass operation as a treatment of obesity. *Ann. Intern. Med.*, 85:97–109.
9. Brill, A. B., Sandstead, H. H., Price, R., Johnston, R. E., Law, D. H. IV, and Scott, H. W., Jr. (1972): Changes in body composition after jejunoileal bypass in morbidly obese patients. *Am. J. Surg.*, 123:49–56.
10. Buchwald, H., Moore, R. B., and Varco, R. L. (1975): The partial ileal bypass operation in treatment of the hyperlipidemias. *Adv. Exp. Med. Biol.*, 63:221–230.
11. Buchwald, H., Varco, R. L., Moore, R. B., and Schwartz, M. Z. (1975): Intestinal bypass procedures. *Curr. Probl. Surg.*:1–51.
12. Buckwalter, J. A. (1977): A prospective comparison of the jejunoileal and gastric bypass operations for morbid obesity. *World J. Surg.*, 1:757–768.
13. Buckwalter, J. A. (1980): Morbid obesity: Good and poor results of jejunoileal and gastric bypass. *Am. J. Clin. Nutr.*, 33:476–480.
14. Buckwalter, J. A., and Herbst, C. A. (1980): Complications of gastric bypass for morbid obesity. *Am. J. Surg.*, 139:55–60.
15. Christakis, G. (1973): The prevalence of adult obesity. In: *Obesity in Perspective*, edited by G. A. Bray, pp. 209–213. D.H.E.W. Publication No. (N.I.H.) 75–708.
16. DeOrio, A. J., and Greenlee, H. B. (1977): Peptic ulcer surgery. *Surg. Clin. N. Am.*, 57:1167–1168.
17. DeWind, L. T., and Payne, J. H. (1976): Intestinal bypass surgery for morbid obesity. Long term results. *JAMA*, 236:2298–2301.
18. Drenick, E. J., Simmons, F., and Murphy, J. F. (1970): Effect on hepatic morphology of treatment of obesity by fasting, reducing diets and small bowel bypass. *N. Engl. J. Med.*, 282:829–834.
19. Drenick, E. J., Bale, G. S., Seltzer, F., and Johnson, D. G. (1980): Excessive mortality and causes of death in morbidly obese men. *JAMA*, 243:443–445.
20. Goldberger, J. H., Chung-Ja, C., Hazard, W. L., Randall, H. T., and Clowes, G. H. A. (1976): Jejunoileal bypass for morbid obesity: Early results and body composition changes in forty-five patients. *Surgery*, 80:493–497.
21. Gomez, C. A. (1979): Gastroplasty in morbid obesity. *Surg. Clin. North Am.*, 59:1113–1120.
22. Gomez, C. A. (1980): Gastroplasty in the surgical treatment of morbid obesity. *Am. J. Clin. Nutr.*, 33(Suppl.):406–415.
23. Griffen, W. O. (1979): Gastric bypass for morbid obesity. *Surg. Clin. North Am.*, 59:1103–1112.
24. Griffen, W. O., Jr., Young, V. L., and Stevenson, C. C. (1977): A prospective comparison of gastric and jejunoileal bypass procedures for morbid obesity. *Ann. Surg.*, 186:500–509.
25. Halverson, J. D., and Koehler, R. E. (1981): Gastric bypass: Analysis of weight loss and factors determining success. *Surgery*, 90:446–455.
26. Heimburger, S. L., Steiger, E., Logerfo, P., Biehe, A. G., and Williams, M. J. (1975): Reversal of severe fatty hepatic infiltration after intestinal bypass for morbid obesity by calorie-free amino acid infusions. *Am. J. Surg.*, 129:229–235.

27. Kannell, W. B., and Gordon, T. (1979): Physiological and medical concomitants of obesity: The Framingham Study. In: *Obesity in America*, edited by G. A. Bray, pp. 125–163. D.H.E.W. Publication No. (N.I.H.) National Institute of Health, 79–359.

28. Laws, H. L., and Piantadosi, S. (1981): Superior gastric reduction procedure for morbid obesity. *Ann. Surg.*, 193:334–336.

29. Lechner, G. W., and Callender, A. K. (1981): Subtotal gastric exclusion and gastric partitioning: A randomized prospective comparison of one hundred patients. *Surgery*, 90:637–644.

30. Lew, E. A., and Garfinkel, L. (1979): Variations in mortality by weight among 750,000 men and women. *J. Chronic Dis.*, 32:563–576.

31. Lindner, P. G., and Blackburn, G. L. (1976): Multidisciplinary approach to obesity utilizing fasting modified by protein sparing therapy. *Obes. Bar. Med.*, 5:198–216.

32. MacLean, L. D., Rhode, B. M., and Shizgal, H. M. (1981): Gastroplasty for obesity. *Surg. Gynecol. Obstet.*, 153:200–203.

33. Maini, B. S. (1977): Surgical approaches. In: *Obesity*, edited by G. L. Blackburn, pp. 40–59. Center for Nutritional Research, Boston.

34. Maini, B. S., Blackburn, G. L., and McDermott, W. V. (1977): Technical considerations in a gastric bypass operation for morbid obesity. *Surg. Gynecol. Obstet.*, 145:907–908.

35. Mason, E. E., and Ito, C. (1967): Gastric bypass in obesity. *Surg. Clin. North Am.*, 47:1345–1351.

35a. Mason, E. E., and Ito, C. (1969): Gastric bypass. *Ann. Surg.*, 170:329–339.

36. Mason, E. E., Printen, K. J., Barron, P., Lewis, J. W., Kealey, G. P., and Blommers, T. J. (1979): Risk reduction in gastric operations for obesity. *Ann. Surg.*, 190:158–165.

37. Mason, E. E., Printen, K. J., Blommers, T. J., Lewis, J. W., and Slom, D. H. (1980): Gastric bypass in morbid obesity. *Am. J. Clin. Nutr.*, 33:395–405.

38. Mason, E. E., Printen, K. J., Hartford, C. E., and Boyd, W. C. (1975): Optimizing results of gastric bypass. *Ann. Surg.*, 182:405–414.

39. Palgi, A., Bistrian, B. R., Greenberg, I., and Blackburn, G. L. (1982): Significant weight loss (>40 lbs) and prolonged maintenance (2–7 years) with medical treatment of obesity. *Ann. Intern. Med. (in press)*.

40. Palombo, J. D., Maletskos, C. J., Reinhold, R. V., Hayward, E., Wade, J., Bothe, A., Benotti, P., Bistrian, B. R., and Blackburn, G. L. (1981): Composition of weight loss in morbidly obese patients after gastric bypass. *J. Surg. Res.*, 30:435–442.

41. Passaro, E., Jr., Drenick, E., and Wilson, S. E. (1976): Bypass enteritis. A new complication of jejunoileal bypass for obesity. *Am. J. Surg.*, 131:169–174.

42. Payne, J. H., and DeWind, L. T. (1969): Surgical treatment of obesity. *Am. J. Surg.*, 118:141–147.

43. Payne, J. H., DeWind, L. T., and Commons, R. R. (1963): Metabolic observations in patients with jejunocolic shunts. *Am. J. Surg.*, 106:273–289.

44. Payne, J. H., DeWind, L., Schwab, C. E., and Kern, W. H. (1973): Surgical treatment of morbid obesity. *Arch. Surg.*, 106:432–437.

45. Peltier, G., Hermreck, A. S., Moffat, R. E., Hardin, C. A., and Jewell, W. R. (1979): Complications following gastric bypass procedures for morbid obesity. *Surgery*, 86:648–654.

46. Salmon, P. A. (1971): The results of small intestine bypass operations for the treatment of obesity. *Surg. Gynecol. Obstet.*, 153:200–208.

47. Scott, H. W., Jr., Brill, A. B., and Price, R. (1975): Body composition in morbidly obese patients before and after jejunoileal bypass. *Ann. Surg.*, 182:395–404.

48. Scott, H. W., Jr., Dean, R., Shull, H. J., Abram, H. S., Webb, W., Younger, R. K., and Brill, A. B. (1973): New considerations in use of jejunoileal bypass in patients with morbid obesity. *Ann. Surg.*, 177:723–735.

49. Scott, H. W., Lew, D. H., Sandstead, H. H., Lanier, V. C., and Younger, R. K. (1970): Jejunoileal shunt in surgical treatment of morbid obesity. *Ann. Surg.*, 171:770–782.

50. Sherman, C. D., Jr., May, A. G., Nye, W., and Waterhouse, C. (1965): Clinical and metabolic studies following bowel bypassing for obesity. *Surg. Gynecol. Obstet.*, 132:965–979.

51. Shizgal, H. M., Forse, R. A., Spanier, A. H., and McLean, L. D. (1979): Protein malnutrition following intestinal bypass for morbid obesity. *Surgery*, 86:60–69.

52. Spanier, A. H., Kurtz, R. S., Shibata, H. R., McLean, L. D., and Shizgal, H. M. (1976): Alterations in body composition following intestinal bypass for morbid obesity. *Surgery*, 80:171–177.

53. Stunkard, A., and McLaren-Hume, M. (1959): The results of treatment for obesity. A review of the literature and report of a series. *Arch. Intern. Med.*, 103:79–85.

54. Van Itallie, T. B., and Burton, B. T. (1979): National Institutes of Health Consensus Development Conference on Surgical Treatment of Morbid Obesity. *Ann. Surg.*, 189:455–457.
55. Westlund, K., and Nicolaysen, R. (1972): Ten-year mortality and morbidity related to serum cholesterol. A follow-up of 3,751 men aged 40–49. *Scand. J. Clin. Lab. Invest.*, 30:1–24.
56. Zelman, S. (1952): The liver in obesity. *Arch. Intern. Med.*, 90:141–156.

Health and Obesity, edited by H. L. Conn, Jr.,
E. A. DeFelice, and P. Kuo. Raven Press,
New York © 1983.

Panel Discussion

Hadley L. Conn, Jr.

*Department of Medicine, University of Medicine and Dentistry of New Jersey,
Rutgers Medical School, Piscataway, New Jersey 08854*

Dr. Conn: Dr. Leibel has presented evidence suggesting that there is a major genetic determinant of the ultimate outcome (degree of obesity) and Dr. Van Itallie has indicated some ways in which the genetic determination might be expressed but apparently not in terms of fat tissue shunting, energy available to fat cells, or in terms of fat cell responses. Even though these aren't the prime defects, is intervention in one or another of these other aspects likely to be useful in the treatment of obesity? Is there any evidence that suggests the fundamental process involved? Is there, for example, a primary defect in cell membrane receptor?

Dr. Leibel: I don't know what metabolic processes ultimately express the apparent genetic contribution to risk of obesity in man. I suspect, however, that the mechanism is not *primarily* located in the adipose tissue. It is much more likely that an individual's susceptibility to obesity is dictated by subtle differences in rates of energy-costly processes such as ion pumping and protein turnover. Adipose tissue morphology is to a large extent only a reflection of long-term energy balance. There are, however, probable differences among individuals in terms of the relative responsiveness (reflected in fat cell hyperplasia) to a given degree of stimulation (e.g., storage of excess calories).

Dr. Conn: Maybe you would like to comment, Dr. Van Itallie, but before you do here is a question that seems related to the previous one. "We have always been taught that weight gain or loss depends on difference between intake and output. If two people expend the same amount of energy, how do you explain the weight gain in one of them, even in the face of larger and more fat cells? Can this all be due to thermogenesis?"

Dr. Van Itallie: We continue our belief in the laws of conservation of energy. But the fact is that there are differences in resting metabolic rate, in physical activity, and in diet-induced thermogenesis that can account for different responses to the same caloric intake, if we are convinced that our measurements are not giving us spurious results. We have to believe that anecdotal accounts of fat people gaining different amounts of weight on the same diet are subject to rational explanation. I would like to comment on the fact that, although I believe that the genetic component of obesity is probably very strong in many instances, the environment in which the individual lives must play an important role in bringing out his/her susceptibility to obesity. We know that one hundred years ago there were far fewer obese people in the United States than there are now. Our diet has changed and our energy expenditure has changed. People who are vulnerable to obesity in a certain environment don't become obese when there is not enough food or the food isn't right. When you live in an environment such as ours, where physical activity is low, the fat content of the diet is high, and the diet is varied and palatable and always available, any genetic susceptibility to excess fat storage will be "exploited" by the environment. I think the relative importance of these two elements, nature and nurture, has to be kept constantly in mind.

Dr. Conn: Dr. Van Itallie, there is a conventional wisdom that timing of food intake is important to weight control. Such wisdom holds that, if a person eats a large breakfast and lunch but a small dinner, he will be thinner than a person who eats little breakfast or lunch but a big dinner and evening snack, providing the total caloric intake is the same. Is there any basis for this conventional wisdom?

Dr. Van Itallie: I don't think there is very much. There was an Australian worker who did some studies suggesting that if the preponderance of the day's calories was consumed in the morning, that somehow would be conducive to loss of weight, or less efficient retention of calories or fat. That work was incomplete and has never been confirmed. So, although I think more research might be done on this subject, there is little evidence to support the suspicion that it matters how you distribute your intake of food during the day.

Dr. Conn: Dr. Kuo, a series of questions are addressed to you. I will try to combine them into two or three. How many calories are offered in your diet, and what do you recommend regarding complex carbohydrates and fiber content?

Dr. Kuo: The diet presented in my chapter is designed to restrict the number of calories but not to require counting calories. As you know, it is very difficult to get patients to count calories each time they eat a meal. It is just impractical. In our program we emphasize restriction of the calorie-dense, simple or refined carbohydrate(sugar)-containing foods and drinks. By adhering to this principle we could achieve good metabolic control of a subgroup of overweight patients with hypertriglyceridemia (very low density lipoprotein elevation). With regard to the fiber content, the total insoluble fibers that we get from a vegetable and fruit are not as beneficial as the more gummy "fibers" such as oatmeal and other cooked cereals. The latter seem to be more effective in the normalization of lipid metabolism. On the question of complex carbohydrates versus the more refined carbohydrates, there has been controversy in regard to the intake of starches versus sugars. It was assumed that the absorption and metabolism of sugars and starches are similar. More recent studies seem to show that complex carbohydrates (starches, for example) do not evoke the same degrees of hormonal or metabolic response that simple carbohydrates (sugars) do.

Dr. Conn: Two people have asked about eggs, so that must be important.

Dr. Kuo: What concerns us is the yolk part of the egg, which is high in cholesterol. An average-size egg contains approximately 250 mg of cholesterol, which is emulsified in phospholipids to facilitate absorption. Egg is a very nutritious food. Its effects vary from one person to another. If one has normal metabolism, I believe that two to three eggs per week as suggested by the American Heart Association provide good nutrition. However, in persons who have abnormal cholesterol metabolism, that would constitute excessive cholesterol intake. By omitting egg yolk, you can lower serum cholesterol concentrations by almost 10%. If you are dealing with patients who have familial hypercholesterolemia, egg yolk has to be very strenuously restricted.

Dr. Conn: You said that you recommend approximately 40% of the calories in the form of carbohydrate and 20% protein, leaving 40% fat. Isn't this high? Even the American Diabetes Association recommends 55% carbohydrate and a substantial decrease in fat. Would you please comment? A related question deals with outcome. When you tell us your results were effective, what do you mean? How much weight did patients lose, how much did blood pressure change, those sorts of things?

Dr. Kuo: As you noticed we have presented a group of patients who are middle-aged, overweight, with borderline disturbances in carbohydrate metabolism. This includes some who gain weight after middle-age probably related to both prosperity and sedentary lifestyle, a major genetic factor combined with environmental and dietary factors. Therefore, in our dietary plan we reduce one major source of calories, i.e., sugars or refined carbohydrates. We achieve the desirable clinical and metabolic effect of the diet without changing too much of its basic nutritional content. It is relatively easy to follow and the results have been good. The clinical outcomes so far are good with respect to weight loss, complications, and control of symptoms. Therefore, the patient has the incentive to continue the diet because most of my patients have symptoms of cardiovascular disease.

Dr. Conn: There are two questions addressed to Dr. Kannel. One asks, "How is it possible to reconcile your statistics on health risk with the assertion of Dr. Ruben Andrus that obesity is not a health risk?" And a somewhat related question: "What about routine screening of triglyceride and high density lipoprotein levels in adult patients?" The questioner quotes a review in the *New England Journal of Medicine*, without precise citation, that expresses doubt of the value of triglyceride screening and finally a Medical Letter in the *New England Journal* commenting on wide discrepancies in HDL values among commercial labs. So in effect the bottom line is, what do you advise the individual practitioner to do when faced with this problem in clinical practice?

Dr. Kannel: Regarding Andrus' assertion that obesity is harmless, I don't think he quite says that. I think what he suggests is that the optimal or ideal weight may be a bit greater than formerly recommended by the insurance industry. I think even the insurance industry statistics now seem to indicate a J-shaped or quadratic relationship at variance with the former concept that the lower the weight the better. Hence, one should not attempt to emulate "Twiggy," as there may be a penalty involved as we do not really know what is going on at very low weights. My view is that if one can be fattened without altering one's lipids, blood pressure, carbohydrate tolerance, and uric acid, it is possibly innocuous. However, I don't think many people can do that. Within the plump American population, there is no question that the fatter one is, the more liabilities one incurs. Remember with regard to optimum weight that one has to define in terms that reconcile both the quality of life as well as quantity. If one lives as long as expected but with gallbladder disease, diabetes, heart attacks, strokes, and heart failure, is the long life worth it?

Dr. Conn: You mean that if you eat rat pellets all your life you may be thin but not happy.

Dr. Kannel: In respect to the triglyceride issue there is great confusion. One thing is clear: Coronary patients have higher triglyceride values than noncoronary patients. It is also true from prospective epidemiologic studies that persons with high triglyceride values develop more coronary disease than those without them. The question is whether the coronary heart disease-related hypertriglyceridemia is fundamental to the atherosclerotic process. The evidence suggests that the other lipid components are more important because, if one does multivariate analysis to assess the net effect of the various lipids after taking the other correlated risk variables into account, there doesn't seem to be much left over for triglyceride. That is, there is an excess risk associated with high triglyceride levels that seems to be accounted for by the lower-than-average HDL values and the greater-than-average degree of obesity and the impaired carbohydrate tolerance that high triglyceride people exhibit.

Dr. Conn: What you might be saying is the reverse of that, that those other three relationships are really a consequence of the hypertriglyceridemia correlation.

Dr. Kannel: Except for the fact that if you change the triglyceride you do not alter the other factors, and if you change the other factors you do alter triglyceride. Furthermore, whereas one can show LDL carrying lipid into the cell and producing atherosclerotic lesions and show HDL removing lipid from tissues, nobody has been able to show triglyceride inducing these things or improving the situation. Solely altering the triglyceride is hard to do. I think that Dr. Kuo is probably correct in noting that triglyceride is carried in VLDL and that VLDL is the precursor of LDL and is therefore involved in the intermediate metabolism of lipids. Triglyceride and VLDL are also strongly inversely correlated with HDL and thus there may be an intermediate metabolic connection. We still have more information to sort out before we can fully understand the role of triglyceride. In terms of risk assessment, however, if we know the HDL level and the total cholesterol or LDL-cholesterol, incidence of atherosclerosis can be predicted quite well. Getting further information on triglycerides for purposes of prediction doesn't seem to provide any additional advantage. Most people with high triglycerides encountered clinically tend to be overweight, diabetic, or use too much alcohol; control of these eliminates the hypertriglyceridemia in two-thirds.

Dr. Conn: The next question is directed to Dr. Van Itallie and other panel members. What are your recommendations for a therapeutic program for adult humans who are more than 150% of ideal body weight?

Dr. Van Itallie: Adult humans who are 150% or more of ideal or desirable weight are severely obese. There are approximately 7 to 8 million such people in the United States, according to the most recent data from the National Center for Health Statistics. In the treatment of those individuals, much attention must be paid to the impairments associated with this degree of severity, impairments through which obesity probably exerts most of its undesirable effects. There are certainly problems such as loss of agility, impaired fertility and menstruation, and susceptibility to accidents that do not necessarily impinge directly on mortality, and thus do not need treatment directly oriented to life span. The people with severe obesity are not a homogeneous group. There are different ways people can become obese. The first step is to try and determine in a given individual, if possible, what the problem is and the extent of its response to treatment. There may be many subtle differences among obese persons that cannot be readily determined. In our own weight control program we use an individualized approach. The first thing that we require of the patient is a strong commitment to lose weight. This requires the obese individual to make a substantial readjustment in life-style and to demonstrate this by many objective means rather than mere vocal affirmation. The obese individual has to accept that obesity is a chronic life-long disease, which is only in remission after weight loss. The basic problem is always present, and self-discipline needs to be maintained constantly by the individual. There is a category of obese individuals who are compulsive overeaters and do not seem to be able in many circumstances to control their eating behavior. Those individuals can be referred to Overeaters Anonymous or a similar self-help group that deals with compulsive overeating. In addition, increased exercise combined with a reshaping of one's whole life-style is an approach that will help the individual to maintain weight loss. His exposure to food is reduced and he can be retrained to choose smaller quantities of less fattening foods. Severe obesity is an extremely difficult problem that requires much effort on the part of both therapist and patient. It is not likely to be successful unless a substantial commitment is made by both parties, and treatment is of prolonged duration. I do not believe that a liquid-protein diet or low-calorie "supplemented fast" of 600 calories or less is the answer to the problem. Patients will lose weight on this kind of diet, but for the most part they regain the lost weight unless at the same time they take other measures that will help them maintain control over their eating and exercise behavior.

Dr. Conn: Is the genetic tendency to obesity in children related to whether the obese parent or parents were of childhood-onset or adult-onset obesity?

Dr. Leibel: I don't know of any study that directly addresses that issue. The study by Charney et al. (1) showed an interactive effect of parental overweight and a subject's weight status in the first 6 months of life with regard to the subject's risk of being overweight as an adult. Individuals achieving a weight above the 75th percentile during the first 6 months of life had a 20% chance of overweight or obesity in adulthood if neither parent was overweight. If at least one parent was overweight, the prevalence of obesity in individuals achieving a weight above the 75th percentile during the first 6 months of life increased to 51%. This was a retrospective study in which the pediatric medical records of 20- to 30-year-old subjects were reviewed. The *current* weight and height of the subjects and their patients were determined by questionnaire or telephone interview. No data were collected regarding the age of onset of obesity in the subjects' parents.

Dr. Conn: It is not clear to me whether you believe that in humans a primary defect is fat cell hypertrophy, which then stimulates an increase in the number of fat cells, or whether the increase in number of cells is wholly independent of any initial increment in adipose cell size?

Dr. Leibel: When an overfed adult rat achieves a persistent large increase in fat cell size, adipocyte hyperplasia occurs in certain fat pads (2). The genetically obese Zucker rat, which displays adipocyte hyperplasia even in circumstances of relative restriction of food intake, only does so in association with the achievement of an enlarged adipocyte size (3). A similar phenomenon has been described in a small number of obese children (4). The evidence thus suggest that, in rodents, hypertrophy to a critical cell size may be a stimulus to hyperplasia. In children, the data are much less extensive, but there is a suggestion that in some obese children there is a triggering of fat cell hyperplasia following the attainment of the upper limit of fat cell size (5).

Adipocyte hyperplasia in the absence of hypertrophy has been recently described in the epididymal fat depot of 6-month-old male Sprague-Dawley rats reared in a 5°C environment from age 28 days onward (6). Whether there are environmental/genetic factors capable of inducing hyperplasia without antecedent or attendant hypertrophy in man, is not known.

Since there is no evidence for preferential shunting of calories into fat in obese individuals, it can be assumed that an individual must be in net positive energy balance for the filling of new adipocytes to occur. Positive energy balance may be due to excessive energy intake and/or enhanced metabolic efficiency. Thus, even if primary adipocyte hyperplasia were a factor in some cases of human obesity, a perturbation in energy balance would still be necessary for the clinical expression of obesity.

Dr. Conn: Can a patient on a very low calorie, modified fast be asked to exercise? If yes, how much exercise should he be asked to perform?

Dr. Vertes: I'm glad that question was asked because the word exercise is improperly used. We are really talking about increased physical activity, not necessarily exercise. Yes, we help the massively obese individual find ways to increase his physical activity in his day-to-day life. In addition, we utilize swimming and walking as major activities in this regard.

Dr. Conn: This query is directed to Dr. Bray. In your 800-calorie per day balanced diet, how much carbohydrate, protein, and fat (in grams) do you prescribe for your patient? What kind of exercise program do you prescribe?

Dr. Bray: We structure our dietary program around the Recommended Dietary Allowances prepared by the National Research Council. This group recommends 0.8 g of protein per kg of desired body weight for both males and females. In practical terms this means that a diet with 70 g per day will meet any individual's needs. Next, I provide a mixture of fat and carbohydrate in which carbohydrate predominates at approximately 50% of the remaining calories, and fat makes up the rest. In applying these concepts for out patients we have constructed as part of the Physicians Diet Plan, a calorie exchange list that allows individuals to obtain the appropriate number of calories from each of the major food groups. In addition, we have rated foods according to their nutritional values.

Dr. Conn: A question directed to both Dr. Bray and Dr. Stunkard. "Could you please comment about forms of treatment for that group of individuals who, despite normal or low weight, have a serious form of eating disorder, compulsive binge-fasting syndrome, vomiting, taking laxatives." That sounds to me like a description of anorexia nervosa, or a variant.

Dr. Stunkard: I think that the question deals with bulimia—binge eating—which can occur with or without subsequent vomiting. It may occur along with anorexia nervosa, but it is a different condition that also affects people of normal weight, and even obese persons. We have experience with that kind of problem and it is a difficult one and one that is growing in prevalence. A certain number of these patients respond to drugs, Dilantin® in particular, which we reported in 1977 (7). Dilantin® may be used as a first line of attack. If it works, it is economical, but often it does not work. Only approximately one-third of bulimics respond to Dilantin®.

The second line of attack is the behavioral approaches that are beginning to be developed. They are still experimental and you really need an imaginative behavior therapist who can construct individualized therapy for bulimic patients. The third line of attack is conventional psychotherapy, which can help people become better adjusted. If they are better adjusted, not so anxious and not so upset, they often can control their binging and vomiting; but it is still not a very satisfactory form of treatment.

A fourth approach is through Overeaters Anonymous (OA), a self-help group that is quite different from others such as Weight Watchers and Diet Workshop. OA does not put much emphasis on weight loss, but instead on controlling personal behavior. It is quite similar to AA, and, in fact, derives from AA. It has the same 10 steps as AA. One summer, I attended several OA meetings. My impression was that a large number of the people at those meetings were binge-eaters and vomiters. If a person is a binger and vomiter, OA can be useful. On the other hand, it is my experience that it is rather hard to get people to go to OA, just as it is hard to get alcoholics to go to AA meetings. Only a fraction of the alcoholics who begin with AA stay with it, but that doesn't mean it isn't worth trying. And it's the same with OA. When it works, it may be through a sort of spiritual approach. If a person will go to one of these organizations, this spiritual approach may offer him as much as anything that we have right now.

Dr. Conn: Do you believe that protein-sparing modified diet programs should currently be supervised only in specialty centers under protocol, or do you believe that general internists or family practitioners can supervise these kinds of therapy?

Dr. Vertes: I think that patients on all very low calorie diets must be closely supervised. There is no question of that. By definition, the patient who needs this kind of therapy has a large amount of weight to lose and probably has medical problems that need careful monitoring. This should be done under medical supervision. I do not believe it has to be done in a medical center. I think it can be supervised by a family practitioner provided he has been trained in proper patient selection and monitoring for the supplemented fast. With this proviso, he can adopt the guidelines of Blackburn and associates, which combine behavioral and dietary approaches. If the clinician is willing to do this, I think the program doesn't have to operate in a center.

Dr. Conn: What are the supplemental diets available in the market called? Is one called Optifast? Where is Optifast 70 obtainable? Where can one read about the entire program? Can it be used on patients who are 40 pounds overweight and cannot lose weight?

Dr. Vertes: Let me reemphasize there is nothing magical in Optifast 70. It is one type of supplement, the one with which we have had a lot of experience. It is made by the Delmark Corporation of Minneapolis, Minnesota, who at the onset agreed with us not to sell this product over the counter nor to physicians who had not been thoroughly trained in its use. At Mt. Sinai Medical Center, we have had more than 3,000 patients on this program. The Delmark Corporation has data on more than 60,000 patients. We know what this supplement can and cannot do. It is Delmark's responsibility to upgrade trace elements to assure purity of the product and to supply us with a proper supplement. The use of this kind of program has been amply reported in the literature. There may be many other supplements that are also valuable, however, I am unfamiliar with their use or manufacture. I have also not seen any clinical data published in the literature and, therefore, I cannot attest to their value. After all, liquid protein was called a supplement.

Dr. Conn: What is the cost for the individual to participate in this modified-fast program? Do third-party insurers pay for this kind of program?

Dr. Vertes: In Cleveland the only cost to the patient that is not covered by a third-party carrier is the supplement. This is considered by the carriers to be food and, therefore, must be paid for by the patient. The rest of the program, including psychiatric consult, laboratory procedures, office visits, and hospitalization—when necessary—are covered as in any other disease. In 1979 we analyzed the cost to a patient of supporting a 250-pound "habit." We found that it was less expensive for him to go on a diet than to purchase the food necessary to maintain that weight.

Dr. Conn: What was the source of the protein? If some of these amino acids and mineral supplements that you use had been added to the collagen liquid protein, would complications including sudden death likely have been avoided?

Dr. Vertes: As far as fortifying collagen with amino acid, this has been tried. In fact, a number of the liquid proteins were fortified with amino acids and that did not eliminate complications. There were many elements missing from the liquid proteins as they were presented to patients in the 1970s. In my opinion the difference between liquid protein and a proper supplemented fast involves not only high quality protein, but proper addition of trace metals and minerals, as well as proper patient selection and management.

Dr. Conn: Would you expect the same symptoms as described in your presentation to occur in a patient on a well-balanced 800-calorie per day diet?

Dr. Vertes: I cannot answer this question from any personal experience. An 800-calorie diet would be out of the range of so-called very low calorie diets and, at least from a theoretical view, there should not be any problems.

Dr. Conn: I was surprised by the lack of discussion of informed consent. Also evidence of follow-up reports to patients, after participating in these studies. Is there not an obligation in these regards?

Dr. Lasagna: In the old days we didn't mention informed consent because we didn't get it and now we don't mention it because we always get it.

Dr. Conn: What benefits does the use of a formula diet confer over the use of animal protein served in its natural form? Wouldn't the presentation of some kind of food during the modified fast help the patient to learn proper eating behavior, thus promoting weight loss maintenance after the termination of the fast?

Dr. Vertes: I think that is an excellent question and a very pertinent one. In our experience, where we used both kinds of programs, we found that the majority of our patients did not want to make any selections or to look at foods. They preferred just opening a package and mixing the contents and not having to measure or deal with ordinary foods. In his program Dr. Blackburn has found that he can handle his patients on natural foods and that these patients can successfully tolerate this regimen. I think one way is as good as the other. If we do start with a formula diet, I think it is pertinent to reintroduce natural foods as soon as possible, since the patient must get used to the concept of eating food. We made this error in the beginning when we kept patients on the chemical formula diet until their weights were down to ideal and then reintroduced them to natural food. It was difficult for the patient to deal with natural foods.

In recent years we have done the following: After the patient has lost 50 pounds on supplement, he is introduced to one natural food once a day. This is expanded to one meal per day that replaces one supplement. Based on the calories required to maintain ideal weight, a regimen is established to include fixed calories (a prescribed diet) and free calories (a diet of choice within specific caloric limits). I think this affords us a better approach to behavioral therapy in these patients. During the course of treatment, the behavioralist educates the patient in two types of caloric intake. The first type represents a life-long basic diet. The regimen of four supplements and one meal is continued until the physician deems it appropriate to replace the supplements with specific foods. The second type, free calories, is restricted only by total number of calories. One advantage to this approach is that the basic diet offers a safety valve to the successful patient if his weight begins to exceed the permitted weight range. By merely eliminating the free calories, the patient will be able to lose the necessary weight without a total change in diet.

Dr. Conn: Perhaps you can answer this question very quickly. Does this type of fast affect menstruation or ability to become pregnant? And, if one does become pregnant under these circumstances, is there an effect on the fetus?

Dr. Vertes: We have had a number of patients who had either amenorrhea or metromenorrhagia associated with their massive obesity that normalized as they lost weight. Although I have no knowledge of the effects of fasting on conception, I do know that a number of individuals became pregnant while they were on the program. We take our pregnant women off the fast because we have no idea what effect it might have on the fetus including whether or not the formula is protein sparing.

Dr. Conn: Do you recommend the same diet proposed here as a modified fast for those patients who need only to lose 10 or 15 pounds?

Dr. Vertes: No, I would not use this method for someone who has to lose only 10 to 15 pounds.

Dr. Conn: Dr. Blackburn, several questions are addressed to you. One of them is: Do satiety mechanisms function appropriately in patients who have had gastric bypass? What happens if the patient grossly overeats?

Dr. Blackburn: I think that modification of satiety is one of the issues yet to be clarified. A rather dramatic result of the gastric bypass is that there is incredible satiety as well as arrest of hunger in these individuals. This occurs practically instantaneously with recovery from the anesthesia. The effect becomes less as people start to be rechallenged by the temptations of the environment, causing them to start to overeat. I am convinced that one of the key compliance consequences of this operation is the rather remarkable satiety result. Earlier gastric distension obviously is going to occur owing to the small outlet in this small pouch. If we make the pouch smaller and still are able to control the outlet, results are improved further. We ascribe that to altered control via the *vagus* nerve. The feedback from the distension on a variety of gastrointestinal-influencing hormones known to be found in the brain undoubtedly plays a key role. We have also learned that we can educate the patients to dietary restraints that tend to prevent overeating and undue stress on the staple line. Will the staple line disrupt to the extent that the patient will suffer morbidity. No, primarily because the weakest point in the whole system is the gastroesophageal sphincter. When this dilates, the patient will vomit from the overeating and we can turn that into a limiting response. Most people do not enjoy vomiting and wish to avoid it So a combination of physiologic, anatomic, and behavioral influences come together to produce excellent compliance in patients who have failed on numerous attempts to lose weight by medical treatment alone. Control of the "hard-core" overeater by this technique is highly promising, as judged by our 30-month follow-up data.

Dr. Conn: I have several questions for Dr. Stunkard, all of which pretty much reflect one issue. "What are the most important components of a behavioral therapy program? Please elaborate on the specific behavioral modification methods. If behavior modification is not just a series of tricks, please specify what you mean. Would you compare behavior modification to psychoanalytic approaches to weight loss?"

Dr. Stunkard: I will try to outline the general features of the program. I can probably best accomplish this by referring you to manuals on the subject. There are at least three suitable ones. Perhaps the best manual is that of Kelly Brownell, obtained by sending $10 to Dr. Brownell at 133 S. 36th St., Philadelphia, PA 19104. There is a book by Mahoney and Mahoney entitled *Permanent Weight Control*, published in 1976 by W. W. Norton. The third manual is one written by James Ferguson, which is especially helpful because it consists of both a therapist's and a patient's manual. If you are thinking of setting up a program, the therapist's manual is a great help in telling you minute by minute what to do as a therapist. This manual is called *Learning to Eat* and you order several patient's manuals for each therapist's manual. Just write to the publisher, Bull Publishing Company, P.O. Box 208, Palo Alto, CA 94302.

The five major components of a behavioral weight reduction program are (1) self-monitoring, (2) stimulus control, (3) changing the act of eating, (4) reinforcement of the various changes in behavior, and (5) cognitive restructuring. Let me describe these components briefly here. They are described in detail, and how to work with them, in the manuals.

(1) Self-monitoring involves keeping very careful track of everything that the patient eats, and the amount of physical activity, preferably using a pedometer for this latter purpose. Just keeping these records seems to cause people to eat less. In fact, there is one theory that these records are so elaborate and time-consuming that they don't give people time to eat.

(2) The second general approach is what is called "stimulus control," trying to control the stimuli that lead to overeating. This includes such traditional elements as elimination of

the sugar bowl, keeping candy off the table, keeping food out of sight, stocking the refrigerator so that it contains primarily foods requiring considerable preparation (frozen foods or foods that need to be heated). The time spent preparing foods interferes with impulse eating. Keep sticks of carrots or celery in the front of your refrigerator so that they are seen first. Stimulus control involves also paying attention to what you eat and not doing things that distract this attention by such activities as watching television. Many people eat and drink while watching television. Under those circumstances, television watching can become the stimulus for eating. The patients break that combination by eating only at one special designated place and focusing on eating. If they put all of their attention on eating and they eat slowly, they will find themselves satiated more readily, and they will achieve better control of their eating.

(3) Becoming more aware of satiety feelings can help patients change the way they eat, and break up automatic chains of stereotyped eating responses. Another way to help gain control of eating is by slowing the rate of eating by such activities as putting the fork down until each bite is chewed and swallowed. These measures bring more attention to eating and help the patient eat less.

(4) Another approach is a reward system, particularly one in which rewards come quickly. For that purpose, we use a point system, gold stars, silver stars, etc. We like to have the reward given as soon as possible after the desired behavior, in line with Skinner's notion that the more prompt the reward, the more effective it is.

(5) Finally, there is a new method called cognitive therapy. It attempts to deal with negative and pessimistic thoughts, thoughts about the futility of dieting, and the futility of weight loss. It stresses the positive aspects, how much your appearance has changed, how much control has been gained over life, and so forth. Thought patterns are stereotyped. Obese persons, for example, tend to have three or four rather standardized thoughts: "Nothing I do works," "I've always been fat, I always will be fat," "It must be my genes." The aim is to devise counterarguments to these. Patients don't really have to believe the counterarguments in the beginning. But as they identify the negative thoughts and practice the counterarguments, they begin to believe the latter. At first, they may believe the negative thoughts 100% and the positive thoughts 0%. As training goes on, however, credence given to the negative thoughts should decrease and the influence of the counterarguments should increase. It is a method devised to give people a sense of control over their life. Empirically, it does seem to make people feel a lot better.

To summarize, the five major components of behavior modification are (1) self-monitoring, (2) stimulus control, (3) changing the act of eating, (4) reinforcement, (5) cognitive change. All five components are delineated in the manuals I have mentioned above.

Dr. Conn: I have asked Dr. Lasagna to look through the series of questions directed to him and to select two or three he thinks most relevant.

Dr. Lasagna: There is a question of what to do with someone who is overweight and may possibly have some degree of hypothyroidism. Is it better to try thyroxin before T_3? My answer is yes if it works, and one might well continue using it.

Would anorexia-inducing drugs be contraindicated in obese diabetics who hadn't responded to various dietary measures? As far as I am concerned, obese diabetics are best treated by weight reduction. Insulin or oral hypoglycemic agents are usually ineffective. If you can't get patients to lose weight without drugs, then the next best thing is to get them to lose it with drugs. I can accept the use of anorectic drugs in obese diabetic patients who cannot control weight through diet alone.

Finally, is there any value to the use of phenylpropranylamine—an over-the-counter preparation? Phenylpropranylamine is a weak anorectic agent, not a placebo. Its use is comparable to the use of Nytol or Sleep-Eze for sleep problems. I feel the same way about phenylpropranylamine as an over-the-counter preparation for people who need a mild appetite depressant. Someone who is looking for a relatively moderate result is relatively safe here. For someone with serious problems, other drugs or measures are needed.

Dr. Conn: I'd like to take this opportunity to thank the audience for their interest and particularly to thank our distinguished and elegant speakers for their comments.

REFERENCES

1. Charney, E., Goodman, H. C., McBride, M., Lyon, B., and Pratt, R. (1976): Childhood antecedents of adult obesity. *N. Engl. J. Med.*, 295:6–9.
2. Cleary, M. P., Vasselli, J. R., and Greenwood, M. R. C. (1980): Development of obesity in the Zucker obese (fa/fa) rat in absence of hyperplasia. *Am. J. Physiol.*, 238:E284–E292.
3. Faust, I. M., Johnson, P. R., Stern, J. S., and Hirsch, J. (1978): Diet-induced adipocyte number increase in adult rats: A new model of obesity. *Am. J. Physiol.*, 235:E279–E286.
4. Hager, A., Sjostrom, L., Arvidsson, B., Bjorntorp, P., and Smith, U. (1978): Adipose tissue cellularity in obese school girls before and after dietary treatment. *Am. J. Clin. Nutr.*, 31:68–75.
5. Knittle, J. L., Timmers, K., Ginsberg-Fellner, F., Brown, R. E., and Katz, D. P. (1979): The growth of adipose tissue in children and adolescents. *J. Clin. Invest.*, 63:239–246.
6. Miller, W. H., Jr., and Faust, I. M. Alterations in rat adipose tissue morphology induced by a low-temperature environment. *Am. J. Physiol. (in press).*
7. Wermuth, B. M., Davis, K. L., Hollister, L. E., and Stunkard, A. J. (1977): Phenytoin treatment of the binge-eating syndrome. *Am. J. Psychiat.*, 134:1249–1254.

Subject Index